Terminal Hope

D1557215

Terminal Hope

What Cancer Taught Me About Living and Dying

Sharon Eagle

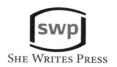

SHE WRITES PRESS

Published 2017
Printed in the United States of America
ISBN: 978-1-63152-288-8 pbk
ISBN: 978-1-63152-289-5 ebk
Library of Congress Control Number: [LOCCN]

For information, address:
She Writes Press
1563 Solano Ave #546
Berkeley, CA 94707

She Writes Press is a division of SparkPoint Studio, LLC.

Dedication

This book is dedicated to a small group of individuals who have quite literally, made my life worth living. First I must thank Lois Davies for her friendship and support for the past 40+ years. She was among the first to visit me in person and share a box of tissues as we absorbed and processed the life-changing news of my cancer diagnosis. For our entire adult lives we have shared life's ups and downs from the day we met on campus at Central Washington University and onward as we married, raised children, struggled in relationships, grew professionally, and developed spiritually. Lois always understood the vital role that hope plays regardless of where we are in life. She was the first to challenge and assist me to identify and clarify my hopes in spite of my diagnosis and prognosis. From the beginning, she gently urged me to write and then gladly read my first attempts, providing loving, honest feedback. I seriously doubt whether this book would have come to fruition without her ongoing encouragement and support.

I cannot imagine my life without my older sister, Stephenie. The important role she has played cannot adequately be expressed in words. Big sis, surrogate mom, close friend, cheerleader, therapist, and so much more. As my first audience, she read through the early attempts and, in spite of a plethora of errors and need for extensive rewrites, she recognized and believed in my vision. Furthermore, she convinced me that it was good enough to actually grow up and become a real book someday. More importantly she and my other siblings, Rick, Roger, and Troy have seen me through the twists and turns, ups and downs, bumps and bruises of life. They have been the support team for the past seven years that every cancer patient should have. Although we all may not have consistently agreed on political or social issues, we always knew without a doubt that we had each other's backs.

I am also grateful to my dear friend Andy McPhee, former Senior Acquisitions Editor at F.A. Davis, my first publisher. He recognized and believed in the writer in me that I wasn't sure existed. Then he took me under his wing and coached me through the process of writing several textbooks for healthcare professionals, an adventure I will always treasure. That experience gave me the confidence to think I might one day be able to write a "regular" book. As we journeyed onward in our lives I've been so pleased that our friendship endured the transition into "retirement" and continues to this day. His was the first professional opinion I sought when the idea of this book crossed my mind. And though he has had no financial or professional gain from this venture, he has consistently encouraged me every step of the way. When I was stuck and undecided between attempting the traditional publishing route (which is notoriously difficult) or self-publishing (which is increasingly popular but fraught with challenges) he pointed me in a third direction toward SWP an up-and-coming hybrid which includes the best features of both words while avoiding the worst perils. It proved to be, for me, the perfect choice.

My mother has always been there for me. Whether here at home where she lives just a hop over the river and twenty minutes away, or out on the road somewhere, I knew I was in her prayers and thoughts. She has always been my role model for what I wanted my retirement to look like. Living independently, working on multiple projects at the same time, especially in the winter. Then when weather permits, packing a small suitcase and traveling around the country to visit relatives and friends in Illinois, Texas, Colorado, Arizona, and Oregon, and all roads in between. Her travels rarely followed a strict schedule, but they were often purpose-driven. There were many nieces and nephews graduating from high school and college each spring, new babies on the way, and a variety of reunions to join in. But of greater importance were those who needed her. Loved ones who were seriously ill, others undergoing surgery, and those who needed an emotional boost. Mom seems to always know who needs her and where she needs to be. She is the glue that holds our extended family together. She shares information among the family that keeps us all informed about how certain ones are doing and who needs some extra TLC. Most of us are poor letter writers (or now I suppose it would be e-mail writers). She serves a valuable role as family communications specialist. Without her, I fear the family groups would fragment and drift apart. She has always filled the role of cheerleader as well. She knows who is working on what projects and makes sure the rest of the family knows about it. She keeps regular prayer lists and prays for those in need. Among some family groups she has been rumored to walk on water. As her daughter I suppose I know her a little too well to share in that belief. However, I know that God uses her quite regularly to convey important information, boost spirits, and help others in ways that most of us will never fully understand. She prays for and shares what little she has with anyone she believes is in need; from public transportation drivers, to family members, to the stranger walking down the street. I have been fortunate enough to call her mother but she is so much more than that. She is also my cheerleader, a prayer warrior for all who know her and many who don't, and an advocate for anyone she believes has been mistreated.

My children; I could easily write an entire book (or several) about each of them but I will try to restrain myself. They have each grown into young adults that I am proud of, people I love to be around. They are parents now and I so enjoy watching them interact with their children. I cannot take full credit for the amazing adults they have become, but if I have had even the smallest influence then I am pleased and honored to know this. When I wonder about what my greatest impact on the world might be, I immediately think of them. They are each unique and different from each other, yet all share certain traits; intelligence, sense of humor, love of family, spirituality, and caring about others. I will probably not know until I've passed on to the afterlife, the full impact they each have had but I am sure there will be positive ripple effects from each of them out into the world and this leaves me feeling grateful.

Contents

Preface: Terminal Hope

I was first diagnosed with stage IV lung cancer in the spring of 2010. I recall a feeling of surreal numbness as I drove home from the clinic while my doctor's words swirled around in my mind, "metastatic lesion", "malignancy", "primary lung tumor", "biopsy" . . . I pushed them away, trying to focus on the road. The last thing I needed now was a car accident . . . Finally I pulled into my own driveway and stumbled through the front door. That's when my knees gave way and I found myself on the floor, my thoughts a jumbled mess. I knew I wanted and needed to pray but felt so out of my depth, drowning, helpless, gasping for air. Finally, I abandoned all pretense of trying to formulate a "normal" prayer and simply confessed to God "I don't know how to do this! It's just too much! Overwhelming! I'm scared and helpless. I can't possibly do this without you!"

As this continued I found certain thoughts going through my mind. "Have I lived my life well? How many opportunities have I wasted? Why didn't I do more to help others? I wanted to make a difference, but did I? I put things off; sometimes the most important things. I always thought I'd have more time. I've been so busy. Too busy. Living my life out of balance. I'm so sorry; for the wasted opportunities, for being so self-absorbed, for making stupid, selfish choices that hurt other people. And now this; cancer. A year to live (if I'm lucky). Not enough time. I've seen cancer deaths. So many times in my nursing career I took care of cancer patients. It was rarely pretty. My patients often suffered things I would never want to face. I did my best to care for them but now I realize I had no clue about how they really felt. How did they do it? It seems to be my turn now and it's so overwhelming. How can I tell my family? How can I possibly tell my mother? She just lost her first-born son (my oldest brother) a few months ago. How can I tell her that she will lose me too? How can I leave my children? The very thought breaks my heart. I don't know how to do this. I don't want to do this. I can't do it without you. Please Lord, show me the way."

I had so many questions and very few answers. Over time, I was able to get basic information from my physician and the oncology nurses. They provided clinical data that helped me understand my treatment choices, medication side effects and the like. Some information was available on the internet. But it could not answer the many personal, emotional questions I had. I felt the need to talk with someone on a similar path.

My family and most close friends were supportive and loving. Some were great listeners. They were caring and sympathetic. Yet they too were struggling to cope with how this would impact their lives. There were times I needed someone who was not quite so close, who was not family. Someone with whom I could voice my distressing fears without worry that I was making them feel even worse than they already did. I needed to feel heard and understood.

Over the next several weeks I looked for a support group but in my small town there were none that fit my need. The closest one I could find was made up almost entirely of breast cancer survivors.

Most were in remission. They were all riding the survivorship bandwagon. They were kind, caring women who invited me to join their club but it did not meet my needs. I know they meant well, but even they refused to discuss the D words (death and dying) and seemed unable to relate to where I was. So next I tried the internet.

After much searching I did manage to find an online cancer support group which even included a conversation thread for people with stage IV lung cancer and a few on the same treatment as I. Finally, just what I needed, or so I thought. Yet after a short time there I found once again that everyone was in survivor mode. Once again it became clear to me in short order that the "D" words were not to be spoken. Everyone was going to survive, regardless of type of cancer or extent of metastasis (spread). To voice thoughts or concerns of anything less was viewed as having "given up." Yet oddly, I noticed that nearly everyone disappeared after three to five years, or sooner. Other than a brief comment about so-and-so having lost her "battle" they were never mentioned again. And rarely did anyone confess that they might have actually died. Denial was pervasive.

Just as frustrating to me was the extent of misinformation being shared. I could appreciate the intent. Most people meant well and were trying to help each other. But as a nurse/nurse educator it deeply concerned me. Some well-meant advice was relatively harmless. But much of it was wrong and some was downright dangerous. I couldn't keep silent and often found myself reverting to my nurse educator role as I attempted to tactfully provide accurate information and where needed, a word of caution. Some members appreciated this and even sought me out (via personal notes or e-mails) for further information and support. But others resented what they perceived to be my know-it-all attitude and became openly argumentative. Worst of all were the ones who didn't even have cancer but were there to sell their magic cures. They professed care and concern but appeared more like vultures circling their prey, out to make a fast buck by taking advantage of people at their most vulnerable. When I confronted a writer (who admitted he was not diagnosed with cancer) about his manipulative words, the site manager responded to me by deleting my entry and scolding me for not being "nicer" to him. In disgust and anger, I promptly deleted my membership information and refused to participate further. Needless to say, I still found myself in search of emotional support and honest conversation. I hoped to be able to share how I really felt and to be honest about my fears and concerns. I hoped I might be allowed to acknowledge the extreme probability that I was going to die in the near future without being accused of being depressed or having given up. I wanted someone who would offer an empathetic ear without all the empty platitudes I was growing so tired of. My continued efforts to find such a group were not successful. I even made discreet inquiries among the nurses and other staff at my medical clinic but none were aware of any support group that met my description. So eventually I gave up on support groups altogether and found myself browsing titles at local book stores. Sadly, I found little there to meet my needs which was somewhat surprising given how prevalent cancer is. Most titles I located were about how to "beat cancer" to become a "survivor" or to "heal yourself" through faith, positive thinking, special diets or the latest magic cures.

So there I was, still in need of a group or even a book that was willing to talk about death and dying, and deal with impossibly painful subjects like how to say goodbye to loved ones, what to expect when dying, and even thoughts about what awaits us after death. I knew I was hardly the first person to face the prospect of dying. Why did it seem to be such a taboo subject? Had the millions, even billions, before me who had died from cancer felt as alone as I did? Did they feel supported? Did they suffer in silence struggling to find their way alone? Or was I really that unique in my need to verbally process everything, even worst case scenarios? Perhaps most people are content to ponder this all quietly to themselves and don't feel the need or desire to talk it out as I did.

Ultimately I had to find my own way. I did this through a combination of personal journaling and frequent conversations with a few close, trusted friends. In particular I found myself spending time in conversation with one of my dearest, long-time friends, Dr. Lois Davies. We met as young adults and have spent our entire adult years as close friends.

As time went by, I outlived my initial prognosis of twelve to eighteen months. And as a result my journal grew to several hundred pages in length. I felt I had been given the gift of time to process my illness-related issues and come to terms with the prospects of dying. Eventually it dawned on Lois and me that between my journal and our conversations, we had created, in very rough form, the very book I had been searching for in the beginning of my journey. We realized it could be a sort of road map, if you will, for how to navigate one of the most challenging times in one's life. With this in mind, she encouraged me to write a book that focused on the major topics of our conversations. There were many recurrent topics that wove their way through our talks and my writings, but the predominant one was hope. I also found myself compelled to read. I was hungry for any information that addressed some of my many questions. I read about death, dying, prayer, trust, faith, angels, hospice care, near death experiences, deathbed visions and the like. I found much of it to be informative and comforting. Therefore, I will share some of what I gleaned with you in the hope that you might also find it of value. Overall my hope is that this book might provide for others what was not available to me when my need was so great. I also hope that healthcare providers who read this will consider the very real possibility that they too may one day be the patient. I pray this has a positive impact as they further consider how they will treat their patients and ultimately how they will prepare themselves for the end of their own journey. It comes far sooner than we expect.

I'm not arrogant enough to think that I have the answers for everyone or that all terminally ill people share the same perspective and needs as I. But if this book helps even a few people to cope more effectively with a fatal diagnosis and to travel their path in less fear and with greater hope, then it will have been worth the effort. This is my intent and my hope.

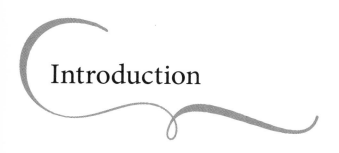

Introduction

You've been diagnosed with a terminal illness. The prognosis is grim. The outcome is certain; doctors say you will die "soon." You may have a few months or only a few weeks. News travels fast among your family and friends. Some pray for a miracle. Other say "there is no hope." Many provide unasked-for advice.

What matters most is how you feel. What you say. Everyone has an opinion, but you are the only one whose opinion really matters. What matters most about hope is if you still have it and what it looks like to you. Does it require potential for a cure? Does acceptance of imminent death mean that you've given up? Or is it still possible, even knowing that you may die soon, to keep hope alive in your heart?

Some believe that death is THE END. Nothing follows. Others believe that death is but a short journey that leads to whatever comes next. What is certain is that life will end for each of us. I've had the privilege of walking beside a number of people and their loved ones as they made their final passage. Each was unique. Each was profound.

Sharon Eagle and I have been dear friends for all of our adult lives. She introduced me to the man who became my husband. Since he was her husband's brother, this made us sisters-in-law when I married him. Sharon and I have loved and supported one another as we've experienced many of life's twists and turns. We raised children, loved and lost friends, loved and lost family, grew spiritually, and shared life's heartaches and joys. We also share a lifelong love of learning. Mine has been in education as a teacher, coach, and administrator. Hers was as a hospital staff nurse and eventually as a nurse educator. I've also had the opportunity to travel alongside and support her after learning she had terminal lung cancer.

Sharon's initial prognosis was for three to twelve months. That was seven years ago. In the first few months I felt compelled to capture the story of her journey. When I first approached her with the idea, she warmly accepted it and we engaged in many lengthy, heart-to-heart conversations. As time passed, weeks turned into months and then years. As always, both of our lives were filled with ongoing surprises and learning opportunities. In the end, Sharon wrote about her journey herself, partly informed by our ongoing friendship and in-depth conversations. I am now privileged to write this introduction.

As a school superintendent in a small rural town, I have had the privilege of sharing many of life's joys and challenges with numerous staff, students, and community members. We've shared the heartbreak of trauma, tragedy, death, and other types of loss. My role has varied according to need—sometimes as a daughter, others as a mother, sister, friend, or colleague. In each case, though our individual paths were unique, we supported one another along the way.

An especially meaningful experience I would like to share is the true story of "Maria." She was an elegant woman who moved to the

United States after retiring as a lead administrative assistant for the director of a large oil firm in Mexico. She left family and friends to marry a gentleman in our small community. She then re-entered the local work force and spent many years supporting migrant and English language learners and their families within our school district. Maria became beloved by all who knew her over the years; working with her was a real joy.

One day I noticed that she appeared unusually weary and frail. I walked her to her office and inquired about how she was feeling. Her honest reply was, "Not well, Mrs. Davies, not well." I encouraged her to take the rest of the day off, go home, and take care of herself. She was reluctant to do so, stating that she still had students to serve that day, but I reassured her that her students would be taken care of and urged her to go on home to rest.

The next day, after being evaluated by her primary care physician, Maria was immediately sent to the regional hospital an hour away. Knowing that she had only a brother-in-law as local family since her husband had passed, I asked two colleagues who lived in the area to check on her. Shortly thereafter they called me with the news that Maria had been diagnosed with an aggressive form of terminal cancer. She was expected to die very soon, with a prognosis of only seven to ten days. The women with her were a bit overwhelmed, wanting to support her but not quite knowing how.

I dropped everything at work and drove to the hospital to be with Maria. After briefly speaking with our colleagues, I entered her room and approached her bedside. I felt so grateful that my lengthy conversations with Sharon had helped prepare me for this and had given me the language needed to talk about hope. Furthermore, I knew that she had limited time and many decisions to make. I gently took her hand and said, "Maria, now that you know you have a terminal illness with only a few days to live, can you describe to me what your hopes are?"

She met my eyes and respectfully said, "I hope to see my husband again. I miss him and look forward to talking with him again."

"Maria, that wish is a clear hope. What do you hope for in the next few days as you prepare to die?"

"Oh, Mrs. Davies, I would like to have hospice," Maria responded in her beautiful accent. "I wish to pass at home. I really liked the hospice nurses and the support they gave me in helping care for my husband as he died."

I was struck by her clarity, elegance, and deep respect in this vulnerable moment.

As I nodded I further inquired, "Maria, what else are you hoping for? How would you like me to share your news at school and with the community?"

"Mrs. Davies, I am so sorry, but I think I need to resign from my job," she said. "I want to spend more time with the students. But I am afraid I won't be able to fit it in." She said this with a serious sigh. I was incredibly touched by her statement and care for our kids.

"Would you like me to help you write a letter to the students?" I asked.

"Yes, I would. Thank you, Mrs. Davies. Writing the letter is an important hope for me. I do not want to be a burden or to impose. It would be very helpful to have you write out my thoughts." She smiled.

"Maria, can you please call me Lois?" I inquired, the cultural formality feeling like a barrier to me.

"Oh no, I could not. I prefer to call you Mrs. Davies. You are my boss," she replied respectfully, with a smile.

"I would be more comfortable with Lois. We are both professional women."

"Mrs. Davies, in my culture you should call me Maria, the students call me Mrs. Smith. I must call you Mrs. Davies. That is what

I am comfortable with. Thank you," she said in a serious and warm manner that implied I shouldn't push further.

I sat down and took paper and a pen to have her dictate her letter to the students and staff. We enjoyed the process of capturing her care and respect for them, her joy in serving and supporting them, and her sadness to have to say farewell in her final letter.

"Maria, who shall I call to share your news and to invite them to come and spend some time with you?" I inquired. "Who do you hope to see?"

"There is no one to call, Mrs. Davies. My friends and family live far away and it is too expensive for them to come," Maria said in a very matter-of-fact and resigned tone.

"Do you have brothers or sisters? Do you have a close friend from over the years?"

"Yes, I have a sister and two brothers. I have a close friend in Wisconsin. But the flights are too expensive and the drive is too far for them to be able to come."

"Do you have any savings or assets?" I asked. "Do you have a will and a plan for how to disperse your things?"

"I do have savings. I do have a will," she told me. "My money will go to my siblings. My home will go to my husband's brother. My things can be shared with anyone who needs or wants them." Again, her practicality and elegant response humbled me. She was clear and able to elaborate her established plans.

"I have a thought," I said. "Would there be enough money to buy a ticket for your siblings or friends?"

"That is a good thought." She paused and her eyes lit up as she reflected on this. "There is enough for a few tickets, but they have busy schedules and I do not know if they would be able to come on such short notice." I could see her hope but also her realistic expectations.

Among a few of us we were quickly able to arrange for hospice care for Maria when she returned home, a private caregiver for several nights until hospice care began, someone to drive her to her follow-up oncology appointment the next week, and travel arrangements for her friend, who would arrive on Monday, and her sister, who would arrive on Tuesday.

Over the next few days, staff members took time to visit and sit with Maria. Many of her students wrote notes to thank her and share their best wishes. Two bilingual educators met her sister at the airport and helped with transportation. Also at Maria's request, they attempted to share certain information about her prognosis that she had not shared. However, the sister was hesitant to believe them and needed to hear it from Maria herself.

From the living room we could hear the emotional conversation between Maria and her sister in her bedroom as she explained that she would die very soon and there was no known cure. After a time her sister came out in tears and asked if we thought anything could be done to treat the cancer and extend Maria's life. We really had nothing to add to what Maria had already told her but we thanked her for coming to spend time with her sister and emphasized how important that was.

As I inquired about any further hopes Maria might have, she mentioned that she had always wished to travel to London. So the next morning, when meeting with her oncologist, she inquired about whether there might be a temporary form of treatment that might buy her enough time and energy to complete this bucket list item. In response the doctor took Maria's hand and tenderly shared her surprise that Maria was doing as well as she was under the circumstances and explained that the trip was not possible. When she commented on how great she looked, Maria responded that most of the time she would have looked better, with makeup on and her hair done more professionally. We all smiled with this elegant lady who was indeed high class. We enjoyed Maria's declaration of how professionally well-kept she generally chose to be. She was disappointed that her trip to London was not possible, but she accepted that the circumstances of her health did not make it a viable option.

After returning Maria home we met with the hospice nurse, who set up a hospital bed in the living room and conferred with us about the use of the prescribed medicines. The nurse then walked outside with me and shared that this was her first hospice case. She was amazed at all we had been able to accomplish in such a short time, from arranging temporary home care and hospice care to bringing Maria's sister and friend there in such a timely fashion. The days ahead were important ones for Maria; by working together we had been able to provide her the loving support she would need, and by gently asking about her last hopes, we had successfully identified the persons and resources needed to help her achieve them.

Over the next several days, Maria moved from her bedroom to the hospital bed. She became less able to chat with us and started to sleep restlessly. Her sister, her friend, and I talked about putting Maria's mind at ease by sharing some very positive stories of her childhood. With the help of an interpreter, her sister told us a very poignant story of a rose garden that had been near their home in Mexico City. She had gone with her sister often to enjoy the beauty of the flowers and the fragrance in the air.

The prognosis of ten days became sixteen. Those who wanted to see Maria and wish her their best had each been able to come by. Her restlessness and quick breathing settled into quiet rest and steady breath. On my last visit with Maria, three days before she passed, she took my hand and looked me in the eye. With a halting voice she said, "Mrs. Lois—I can call you that now—thank you for walking with me as a friend. I am so pleased that my friend and sister came to hold my hand. I loved the letters from the children. They know that I would have come to school to be with them if I could have. I am thankful and at peace. This has been a good life."

I was not with Maria when she took her last breath, but both her sister and friend made a point of sharing with me what those moments were like. Her friend told me firsthand and her sister shared with translation help, and it turned out they shared the same story. They both had sensed the fragrance of roses shortly before Maria took her last deep breath and for several moments following. They both were calmed by the fragrance, and neither one was able to tell the other of this shared sensation at the time. They hugged and cried when they heard each other's tale. Imagined or real, they had shared the same image and sensory experience in spite of the language barrier between them.

While not every passing is as gentle as Maria's, the remembrance of those days seems a fitting introduction to the chapters that follow. The title of this book, Terminal Hope, came directly from those days spent with Maria. My conversations with Sharon led me to ask the questions that set the tone for my conversations with Maria.

Will each of us find the same peace that Maria, her sister, and her friend found in our own journeys of transition? Will the insights Sharon has gained from her journey bring similar insights for us as we each travel our own path and let go of those who pass before us?

Each day is a gift that holds more meaning for me now. The extra days Maria enjoyed, the extra years Sharon has been able to share. And the fact that I now am the survivor of a traumatic brain injury sustained during a major "nonsurvivable car accident." These each add new depth to the meaning of my days.

Lois Davies

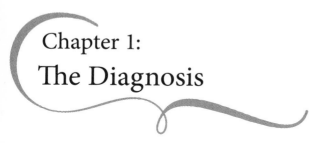

Chapter 1:
The Diagnosis

"Seeing death as the end of life is like seeing the horizon as the end of the ocean."[1]

"Promise me you won't give up." I heard my brother's voice through the heavy darkness of a pervasive nausea unlike anything I had ever experienced before. All I wanted to do in that moment was close my eyes and escape. Talking required too much effort and I didn't want to think, or feel, or give in to any of my senses. It was all too much. I had taken a lorazepam in hopes of escaping into sleep but it wasn't quite enough. I should have taken two but now I didn't have the strength or energy to move, let alone reach for another pill. I didn't know it was possible to feel nausea this profound, this pervasive, in every cell of my body. I remembered once, years ago, my mother describing a nausea so intense that she couldn't even vomit. I didn't know how that was possible. But now I understood. In the past when I vomited I typically felt better, at least for a little while. But this wasn't just in my stomach. I felt it in every part of my body. I felt as if I'd been poisoned and left to die. But then the thought occurred to me, I *had* been poisoned. After all, that's what chemotherapy is. Poison. The hope is that it will be more toxic to my cancer cells than my healthy cells. But right now I wasn't so sure. It felt like all my cells had been poisoned and were slowly dying. It reminded me of the worst hangover I'd ever had (which was pretty bad) but then multiplied by a thousand. I was powerless against it. As another wave of intensely overwhelming nausea came on I managed to slip away into a fitful sleep, futilely hoping I wouldn't wake up until it had all passed.

The next week was a continuous battle. All I recall is a strange sense of darkness interrupted by waves of nausea, and trips between bed and bathroom. I sipped liquids along with an occasional bite of whatever was put in front of me although eating was the last thing on my mind. My mother and daughter were trying so hard to make me feel better, so I forced myself to take tiny bites so I could see the look of relief on their faces.

As soon as they left the room I put the food aside, forced myself to swallow more liquid, and then tried to sleep.

Being a nurse, I was foolishly confident that I could monitor my own fluid volume status. I was peeing often enough and it was a normal light yellow color, which is one of the signs of normal hydration so I thought I was okay. But I was too fuzzy-headed to think clearly or I would have realized that there wasn't nearly enough fluid going in to account for the fluid going out. As the fog of nausea and darkness slowly began to lift I realized that something wasn't right. Although I was feeling better in some ways I was actually feeling worse in other ways. As I thought about it, the image of a wilted, dying plant came to mind. That's when it finally occurred to me to weigh myself. As a nurse I'd often weighed my patients on a daily basis, to watch for increased fluid gain. Less commonly, daily weights can be a useful way to monitor for fluid loss as well. So I staggered across the hall to the bathroom and stepped onto the scale.

"That can't be right," I thought. I weighed myself twice to be sure. In the past week I had lost fourteen pounds. I'm not a large person. Even with shoes on I can barely claim to be five feet tall. Losing this much weight wasn't possible even when I tried hard to do it. That's when I realized how severely dehydrated I was. Somehow I communicated this with my daughter (also a nurse) and she quickly bundled me up and took me to the oncology infusion room at the clinic. I don't recall the numbers but my heart rate was pretty high and my blood pressure was pretty low with a significant postural drop. This means that as I changed position from lying to sitting to standing my heart rate rose higher while my blood pressure dropped lower; a sign of significant dehydration. It took three liters of fluid (slightly more than three quarts) to normalize my vital signs. This left me feeling quite a bit better. The image of the plant came to mind again; but this time it was upright, looking relieved and healthier. Someone had finally given it a drink. Lessons learned: the chemo had an unexpected, strong dehydrating effect on my body, and when I am ill I'm a lousy nurse.

I returned home and crawled back into bed. Although I felt better with more fluid on board, I still felt the aftereffects of two weeks of radiation and a round of chemotherapy. Essentially I felt generally lousy but did not threaten to pass out each time I climbed out of bed; which was a decided improvement.

Unable to sleep, I lay there pondering events of the past several months. I knew I was in trouble the day Lilly called me at work with instructions to see my doctor that same afternoon. Lilly was the primary nurse who worked with Dr. Stevens, my family doctor. She said that he wanted to go over some recent test results with me. I'd had two tests done that week; a chest CT scan three days prior and a lumbar (low back) MRI completed just that morning. A CT (computerized tomography) scan is a radiological procedure that uses computer processing and multiple x-rays taken from numerous angles to create a cross-sectional image. An MRI (magnetic resonance imaging) is a radiological procedure that uses a magnetic field and radio waves to create detailed images. I expected the CT to reveal nothing but healthy lung tissue. I expected the lumbar MRI to show a mild increase in the bulging of a lumbar disc. It had first acted up when I was just fifteen years old and had bothered me occasionally ever since. I was now fifty-three and had recently been feeling more persistent low back pain than before. However, I had recently been to my doctor for this problem so I was puzzled as to why this situation warranted yet another personal visit.

As a nurse, I knew that good news was typically given to patients via mail or over the telephone while face-to-face meetings were generally reserved for dispensing bad news. So why did they need to meet with me in person? What could be so awful about my lumbar disk that warranted a face to face visit? I wanted to ask Lilly what was going on, but as a nurse, I knew that she couldn't and wouldn't tell me. So I didn't pry and resigned myself to waiting until my appointment.

Two hours later Dr. Stevens greeted me warmly as always, but with a more serious demeanor than usual. Having given bad news before, he knew it was best to get right to the point. So he brought the MRI image up on the computer screen in the exam room where we could review it together privately. As expected, my lumbar disc looked a bit worse than before, which might explain the recent worsening of my low back pain. But then Dr. Stevens showed me the quarter-size spot glowing ominously nearby. This "abnormal lesion," he explained, had the appearance of a "malignant (cancerous) mass" that had likely metastasized (spread) from elsewhere in my body.

I was dumbfounded. Other than the annoying, periodic, low back pain, I'd always been pretty healthy. In fact, I'd often said I expected to live well into my eighties since all of my grandparents had lived long lives and both of my parents were still alive. In fact, both were in their eighties and were still active, lived independently, and were reasonably healthy. My mother frequently traveled around the country visiting friends and relatives and I had expected to follow her example when I retired.

So where had this mysterious lesion come from? In truth, I knew the answer but had literally put it out of my mind. The other test I'd had that week, the chest CT scan I expected to come up clean, in fact had showed a lesion that had been noted three months previously at the hospital, also by CT scan. As incomprehensible as it might seem now, I had actually forgotten about it. At the time, the radiologist had specifically said that it did not look like cancer. We were only repeating the CT now as a "normal medical precaution." I was so sure the lesion would have healed by now that I very nearly cancelled the follow-up CT, believing it to be pointless. Apparently I was wrong.

How had all of this happened? Three months earlier I had noticed a deep aching sensation in my left chest and shoulder. I'd been in bed, ready to go to sleep. Like most healthcare providers I was much more comfortable being the nurse than the patient and the last thing I wanted to do at that hour was go to the doctor. The medical clinic would be closed which meant going to the hospital emergency department. I was way too comfy to consider dressing and driving over there. Besides, the pain wasn't that bad. I was sure it was just one of those mysterious aches and pains that become more common with aging. So I took some acetaminophen (Tylenol) for pain, a diphenhydramine (Benadryl) tablet to help me sleep, turned out the lights, and went to sleep.

The next morning the pain was forgotten. But as the day wore on I noted its return. Feeling that I was too busy to be sick, I convinced myself it would go away as it had before and I dove head first into my work. Being a nursing educator at the local community college was a demanding, sometimes stressful job, but one that I loved. So it was always easy to immerse myself in my work and forget about everything else.

At home later that evening I noted the pain was still present and had actually worsened. This time, in addition to the two extra strength acetaminophen I also took a naproxen (Aleve) tablet, all without relief. I lay there pondering the matter, and like many healthcare givers are prone to doing, I began trying to diagnose myself. I considered the most serious possibility, a heart attack. But considering my medical history I quickly discarded that thought. After all, I had no known heart disease, had never smoked, had normal blood pressure, and was still considered "relatively" young at 53. I had no chest pressure, no nausea, no shortness of breath or sweating.

Next I considered costochondritis (an inflammation around the sternum and ribs), or a pulmonary embolism (PE, a clogging of the lung blood vessels). Based on my risk factors and symptoms, I ruled out the former but remained suspicious of the latter.

I still wanted to chalk this up as one of the aches and pains of aging, but a little nagging voice in the back of my mind wouldn't let me do so. As I thought it over I realized that the last thing I wanted was to collapse in front my nursing students the next day with a massive PE. I needed to be up early so I could go to the hospital to teach and supervise my students and it was already after midnight. Clinical days were fun, but also busy and physically and mentally demanding. I owed it to my students to be at the top of my game. They would be scattered all over the hospital taking care of their chosen patients. As usual, I would put a lot of mileage on my white sneakers as I checked on each of them, answering questions, coaching them through procedures, giving tips on performing physical assessments, administering medications, and documenting care, to name just a few of their daily chores.

As I lay in bed pondering my options the pain continued to worsen. Should I just try to sleep and hope for the best? Should I seek medical care at this late hour? Should I cancel clinical (which meant calling and waking each student at this ungodly hour)? Unlike with some other jobs, nursing educators are truly indispensable. There is rarely anyone to step in at the last minute if an instructor falls ill. If I couldn't be there, then neither could my students. And scheduling a makeup day was nearly impossible. I didn't want the students to suffer because of my health issues. Finally, I considered how I might advise anyone else in the same predicament. That's when the answer became obvious, though unwelcome. I sighed deeply, got out of bed, dressed and went to the hospital emergency room to be properly evaluated by a physician.

After collecting my medical history and performing a physical examination the ED doctor concluded (as I had) that I might have a pulmonary embolism. To gather more information, he ordered a D-dimer test which measures fibrin, a substance released into the blood as clots dissolve. An elevated level indicates possible presence of blood clots and my level was above normal. (Much later I learned that an elevated level might also indicate cancer).

While the D-dimer is helpful in ruling out the presence of clots, it is not conclusive for confirming their presence. Nor does it indicate where any clots might be located. Therefore, a pulmonary (lung) CT was required. But the results were a bit puzzling. It revealed a small "mass" in my left upper lung, near the aorta (largest artery exiting the heart). The radiologist said he was confident it was not a tumor and was benign (noncancerous), although he wasn't sure just what it was. After considering my risk factors for cancer, which were pretty much zero, the ED physician finally diagnosed me with atypical (unusual) pneumonia and sent me home with a prescription for pain pills and antibiotics. He advised me to follow up the next week with my primary care doctor. This plan seemed reasonable to me and by the time I met with Dr. Stevens my symptoms had completely resolved. Therefore, the diagnosis made sense and the treatment seemed to have worked.

I was advised to follow up three months later with a repeat chest CT, just to be sure the mass had completely resolved. Though it seems foolish now, at the time I didn't give it another thought. I was sure that whatever it was had gone away.

So now here I was, off work, home in bed, hung over from chemotherapy. Not exactly the big trip to Australia I'd planned for my summer. I had saved money and gotten special permission to begin my end-of-summer break early so I could spend several weeks visiting my son (Brad) and his family in Queensland, Australia. I'd only been there twice in the eleven years he had lived there and was anxious to see him and his family and see more of the country. Now those plans were on hold.

As I lay in bed I grabbed my laptop and opened to the journal I'd started the day before after returning home from the clinic. In the past, when dealing with adversity, I'd found writing to be therapeutic. If there was ever a time I needed therapy, it was now.

Journal May 2010
Wakeup Call

All the way home from the clinic, the Tim McGraw song "Live Like You Were Dying" kept going through my head.[2] It's a great country song about not taking life for granted, but most of us do. I'm as guilty as anyone. I've spent so much of my life focused on the future, achieving the next goal. Yet now I find myself evaluating my life and asking whether I've lived my life well. Have I made a difference in the world or has my focus just been about me? I think I may have made a useful contribution here and there. But I'm also sure I've wasted time, energy, and resources on things that really don't matter.

Yesterday I had a huge wake-up call. I probably have cancer. I'd always wondered how I might feel if I received news like this. My current fears have to do with how this will impact my loved ones. We lost my oldest brother a few months ago. Then my aunt just recently underwent chemotherapy and surgery for breast cancer. It's been a hard year for my mother. I'm not sure she could withstand losing another child. It's every parent's worst nightmare to lose even one child; regardless of age. Now she must face the prospect of losing a second. I'm also concerned for my siblings. They (and I) lost a brother just a few months ago. Even though we all believe we will see him again, the separation is so painful. Something about knowing I won't see someone again in this life makes it feel unbearable. Yet now I suddenly find myself thinking that I may see him sooner than I'd anticipated.

What grieves me most is the thought that I might not be here to help my children when they are going through life's painful times—that I might not be here when they need me. That's a mother's job you know. And my purpose and my joy; to help my children through the tough times and to share in the joys of their good times. I want to do both. Right now my greatest fear is that I may not be around to do either.

By the way, I've never even smoked. How ironic is that? I've only had slight exposure to secondhand and no industrial exposure that I know of. There are no real cancer risks in the family. So it's all a bit weird. It's the one thing that makes me occasionally think that maybe it's not cancer after all—my risk factors are so minimal. All things considered, I've lived a pretty clean life. But then as I've often said to others, "Life's a terminal condition. Ain't none of us getting outta here alive."

Every nurse knows that a diagnosis of cancer isn't official until a tissue biopsy is performed. At first I was terrified of having to undergo a biopsy of the primary tumor in my left lung. The tumor is so close to my aorta that it is unclear whether the aorta might actually be involved. And since the aorta is the largest artery in the body and exits immediately from the heart, I didn't relish the idea of a scalpel or even a needle coming anywhere near it. So as weird as it sounds I was actually somewhat relieved to have the lesion on my sacrum because that meant they could biopsy it instead (even though having the lesion there is what earned me "terminal" status). Like I said, weird. Feelings don't necessarily make sense.

Even so, when it came time for my sacral biopsy I found myself feeling nervous. I had assisted a physician with a sacral biopsy once in the hospital. Even though we pre-medicated the patient with morphine, and he never complained, I could tell that it was still painful. To poke through the hard outer layer of the bone requires a great deal of pressure and use of a tool called a trocar. The best description of a trocar is to say it looks like an extremely large, extra strong needle with a very sharp tip. And when I said that it requires a great deal of pressure, I wasn't kidding. I recall watching the physician stand on her toes so that she could use her body weight to help push the trocar through the tough outer layer of bone.

Journal June 2010
Biopsy

I survived today. As is often the case, the worst part was the anticipation. Reality came crashing in as I lay on the CT table, IV fluids going, and various technicians and the radiologist around me. I found myself fighting to hold back tears; partly due to fear, but mostly from just feeling overwhelmed.

Talk about a reality check. I was silently praying and I knew other people were too but it still felt very scary. Fortunately, that was when they gave me some great drugs that helped me relax. They melted away the fear and alleviated most of the pain. It took about forty-five minutes with various scans and a number of "sticks." They covered me with sterile drapes including one over my head. This allowed me to close my eyes and feel myself bathed in a comforting blue light. I felt God answering prayers in that moment and I survived it much better than I feared I would. There was some pain after. But fortunately the radiologist had injected a large amount of local anesthetic which took several hours to wear off. I only needed one pain pill in the recovery room which worked well. So now, five hours later, sitting on my sofa, I feel pretty ok.

A FEW DAYS LATER...

I met with Dr. Stevens today to get the biopsy results. The sacral lesion is cancerous—the specific type is adenocarcinoma that has metastasized (spread) from the lungs.

Surreality

Hearing that I had terminally advanced cancer was a surreal experience. It took quite a long time for it to sink in. I've always been a realist and never expected to live forever. Even so, having cancer was a difficult concept to wrap my brain around. The practical voice in my brain was saying things like, "You knew it had to happen sometime. Did you think you were gonna live forever? At least now you know how you will die." At the same time the other voice in my brain kept rejecting the entire notion that I might really have cancer and was thinking of the many things left on my to-do list. Besides, cancer is something that other people get. The mental exchange that began that day was to continue for many months, stirred up anew each time another reminder was thrust on me. Little things like the nurse handing me the "Cancer Patient" binder, and me nearly handing it back to her thinking she was mistaken. She couldn't have meant it for me. Additionally, I began to realize with some surprise that the many cancer ads on TV were, to some extent, now talking about me.

Telling Others

One of the things that made my cancer diagnosis feel more real was having to tell others about it. I've heard of others who kept their diagnosis a secret and continued their lives "normally" for as long as they could. I'm not sure how they did it.

I am not one of those people. I have a fairly large family and most of us are verbal processors. This means that we talk a lot. It helps us to think things through, fully understand them, and ultimately cope with them. Even so, telling my loved ones about my cancer diagnosis was one of the most difficult things I've ever done. I remember thinking that I just couldn't make the words "I have cancer" come out of my mouth. I couldn't bear to see the looks of shock, disbelief, and pain that I knew would register on their faces. I couldn't bear to be the cause of the grief, pain, and distress I knew this would bring into their lives. I found myself actually more worried about my family, especially my children, than I was about myself. I wasn't afraid they couldn't handle it; because I knew they could, if they had to. But I didn't want them to have to. I'm the mom and I'm the nurse. I'm the care provider. I'm the one that's looked after them. As busy as I always was, they knew I was there for them. I was the one who kissed their boo-boos when they were small and I was still the one they called on for medical advice, general support, and the special love only a mother can give. The idea of possibly not being here for them one day, when they are in pain, was, and still is, the most difficult thing for me.

The first person I told was my daughter. She knew I had been to the doctor but didn't know why. Yet she took one look at me and knew something was up. As soon as I mentioned the CT and MRI findings she somberly said, "You have cancer." It was a statement, rather than a question. All I could do was nod my head. We hugged and cried, and she promised she would be with me every step of the way. She is a nurse and understood the significance from the very beginning. She was also (thankfully) one of the few people to not immediately jump on the "Think positive! Believe for a miracle!" bandwagon. She knew the odds and she knew that I did too. Yet in her own quiet way, she has been my rock; the most amazing and supportive person and most loving daughter and friend I could ever have asked for. She bore the burden of keeping this secret with me for the following two weeks while I awaited final confirmation via PET scan and bone biopsy. It was a very long two weeks and it was difficult to pretend everything was normal. However, I didn't want to break news of this sort unless I was one thousand percent positive it was accurate. During this time the pragmatic nurse part of my brain knew what the final test results would be, but the human side of my brain was still holding out faint hope that there had been a mistake of some sort. But this was not to be. The PET scan indicated malignancy in my lung and sacrum both. The biopsied tissue from my sacrum confirmed that the cancer there had spread from the primary lung tumor.

As hard as it was for her, my daughter helped me tell the rest of the family. Both of my sons lived out of town and I knew I wouldn't be seeing either of them for quite some time. So even though it was less than ideal, I had to tell them by phone. Yet when we called my middle child, Brian, I couldn't get the words out. I could only sit with my daughter's arms around me as I cried while she told him the news. Then she sat with me as I called my sister Stephenie who lives in the Mid-West. Steph and I have always been quite close and she was devastated by the news, believing since she is the older one, it should be her, rather than me with the cancer. So typical. My big sis had always looked out for me and our other siblings. She was our surrogate mom when our mother was out of the house. I suppose in her place I would feel the same way. Yet I told her that I wouldn't wish this diagnosis on anyone, least of all her. And that is true enough. So we cried together on the phone and promised to get together soon.

Next, Nicole helped me contact my two brothers who live nearby. We asked one of them to pick up my mother and meet us at the other one's house. Of course they sensed that something was up, but followed my wishes without question. It was important to me that my mother not be alone when she heard the news. I knew my brothers would be upset but would be okay. However, I was worried about her and wanted her to be with family when she got the news.

Later that same evening I was able to reach my oldest son by telephone. He has lived some 10,000 miles away in northeastern Australia since 1999.

Brad has a sharp wit and fun, playful sense of humor. These features draw others to him. He is also analytical and sometimes controlling. Such qualities make him a natural leader and others instinctively look to him for advice and guidance. Examples include being the "rules master" of any type of game, (which also brings out his competitive nature), leading outdoor activities with his siblings and cousins and eventually becoming a youth leader at his church. These qualities also impact his decision-making process. With any big decision he carefully gathers all relevant data and may spend hours poring over details. Only then does he make up his mind. This is a strength that usually protects him from impulsivity and rash decisions. Once he has made a decision, his course is set and little can deter him. An example is when, at the age of nineteen, he decided to leave college, move to Australia and join Youth with a Mission (YWAM), to become involved in Christian missions work. While he hoped for his father's and my blessing and support, he was determined to go regardless.

During his teen years, I noticed that he also had a tendency to sometimes be harshly critical of others and insensitive to their feelings. This was not intentional. In fact, he seemed completely unaware until I tried to bring it to his attention. But by then it was already a firmly ingrained habit. Once he reached the conclusion that something was illogical (stupid) he felt compelled to share his insights with others whether they wanted him to or not. I firmly believe he meant well but was unaware of how cutting his words could be and that he sometimes left wounded people in his wake. These same dynamics had been largely responsible for the failed relationship between his father and me. So my greatest concern was that he might repeat his father's mistakes and sabotage any future efforts at developing and maintaining a significant relationship.

Though I resisted his decision to remain in Australia as a permanent resident, I must admit that his time among the YWAM community was an answer to some of my prayers. Each time I visited with him over the following years I noted significant changes in how he interacted with others. The harsh, critical side of his nature was disappearing, leaving a certain softness in its place. He was becoming more considerate and more sensitive to others. Put simply, he was becoming the best version of himself. It is a joy now to watch him interact with his wife in a loving and respectful manner and treat his four boys with more patience and gentleness than I would ever have imagined.

There's never an easy way to share news like mine, but understanding my son's personality style was helpful. I knew what he would need most was data and time to process. So I honestly shared my diagnosis, the significance of stage IV cancer, how it most likely had spread from my lungs to my lower back and my grim prognosis. I shared as much detail as I could. But I let him pull it out of me at his own pace by asking a question, pausing to think it over, then following with another question and so on. He did not cry and expressed little emotion. But I did not expect him to. Fortunately, I understood that his analytical brain was working overtime trying absorb and make sense of it all. I knew the emotion would most likely follow later and be expressed privately. In the days and months to follow, when others asked him how he was doing his typical response was that "Mom is handling it well, and so we are too." It was so good to know that by coping as positively as I could, I was helping my children do the same.

I most dreaded telling my mother because she was still reeling from my oldest brother's death just six months prior. Mom is a woman of faith and prayer. She is also a worrier though she usually denies it. She has a tendency to identify and support whomever she believes to be the underdog in any given situation and will quite literally give away what little she has to anyone whom she believes needs it more than she. She is the emotional caretaker of her family and on many occasions has gone to stay with, and care for, a relative or friend who is ill or recovering from surgery. She also has a habit of making incorrect assumptions and then overanalyzing a situation or innocent comment until she reaches odd conclusions without ever verifying her initial assumption. This sometimes leads to confusion and misunderstandings. But in spite of her quirkiness, she is beloved by most everyone who knows her.

Since my brother's death, mom's behavior has been somewhat unpredictable and fluctuates between extremes of "I know he is in a good place and is happy now" to literally stamping her feet and swearing (and she is not the swearing type). She was angry for a very long time, mostly at God I think, but seemed not to feel okay admitting it. It worsened after my diagnosis. She had so much anger she didn't know how to express yet was unable to cry for a long time. Consequently, she vented her anger at whomever was close at hand, usually her remaining children. We understood and empathized. Yet we were all hurting too and trying to support her while dodging her angry comments was not easy.

I know her anger was a mask for her pain. Watching her oldest son die hurt her deeply in a manner I can only imagine. And, now watching me go through this and feeling helpless to fix it further deepens her pain. Her early comments about how God would surely "perform a miracle" by healing me reflected her denial of my prognosis. Later, she took the improvements in my CT and bone scans to be evidence of my healing. Though I repeatedly attempted to gently speak the truth, she wasn't ready to hear it. However, over time I believe she has slowly let it sink in. Faith is never a perfect thing, but she does have faith and she is stronger than she gives herself credit for. Her anger is slowly dissolving and she seems to be more at peace. This tells me that she is coping better than before and possibly coming to accept the inevitable. Ultimately she copes for the same reason we all must. She simply has no choice.

As for telling the numerous other people in my life, including the students I cared so much about, it was just too difficult to do it all myself. I still felt overwhelmed and, once I began treatment, simply did not have the physical, mental, or emotional energy required. Each time I shared my news with someone I found it to be a bittersweet and emotionally exhausting process. For these reasons, I gave my family, close friends, and nursing faculty permission to share my news with whomever they deemed appropriate. There are times when the local grapevine serves a purpose and for me, this was one of them. It was simply a relief to not need to tell everyone myself.

Chapter 1 Notes

1. Found at several web sites including the following: http://www. quotes.net/authors/David+Searles (accessed 3/25/2017).

    Also found, a quote by Mr. Searls at several sites including his own (davidsearls.com) in which he denies authoring said quote. In his own words "Here's what drives me crazy: That quote attributed to me—"Seeing death as the end of life is like seeing the horizon as the end of the ocean"--is great. It's powerful. It's catchy. People love it. And it's not mine." His theory is that there may be another author by the same name who may have authored it.

2. Tim McGraw, written by Tim Nichols and Craig Michael Wiseman. "Live Like you Were Dying," in Greatest Hits, Vol. 2 CD, Curb Records, August 24, 2004.

Chapter 2:
Treatment, Side Effects, Complications, and Other Fun Stuff

The chemotherapy was very peculiar, something that makes you feel much worse than the cancer itself, a very nasty thing.[1]

As soon as my diagnosis was confirmed I was scheduled to begin radiation. I was given a choice between two or three weeks, five days a week. The doctor recommended the two week course since I was "young and healthy" and could handle the stronger dose. I didn't know any better so I agreed.

JOURNAL JUNE 2010
RADIATION THERAPY

I started my radiation treatments just over a week ago. It was quite easy at first. I don't feel a thing during the treatment and it's not scary. I simply lay on a hard "table" while a huge radiological machine rotates around me making an on/off buzzing sound. The daily treatments are very short—maybe

5 minutes altogether. Side effects began around the fourth day which includes stomach discomfort and diarrhea. So far it is manageable.

Deep Vein Thrombosis

A deep vein thrombosis (DVT) is a blood clot in one of the deep veins, most commonly in the lower legs. If it becomes inflamed with redness, pain, and edema (swelling) then it is called thrombophlebitis. It's not always clear what causes them but a minor leg injury can do it. Risk factors include prolonged sitting or standing, varicose veins, cancer, and elevated platelets or red blood cell levels. Treatment involves anticoagulant medication. A dangerous complication of DVT is pulmonary embolism (PE) which can be fatal.

Journal June 2010
DVT

I noticed a deep, painful aching in my left calf sometime last week which worsened a great deal over the weekend. I nearly went to the doctor on Monday but as I had an appointment set for Tuesday morning I decided to tough it out another day. My leg appeared normal so my oncologist didn't share my concerns. However, I could barely walk from the pain, so I was relieved when he ordered a Doppler study "to be sure." The test confirmed the presence of two large clots in my lower left leg. Normally he would have started me on anticoagulants (blood thinners) immediately. However, I was scheduled for a surgical procedure the next day. Beginning anticoagulants beforehand would greatly increase the risk of excessive bruising and bleeding. So it was delayed until afterwards.

The Power Port

The following day I underwent surgery for Power Port placement. This is a long, fancy sort of central intravenous line. The injection port is implanted beneath the skin, but on top of the muscle, on the left or right upper chest wall. It is threaded to the "entryway" of the heart. There are many other types of central lines and by the time you read this there are likely to be new variations. The purpose of the Power Port is to provide intravenous access to a large, centrally located vein that can tolerate the toxicity of chemotherapy in a way that smaller arm veins cannot. It can also be used for blood draws and infusion of intravenous medications and fluids. This helps save the patient, in this case me, from repeated arm sticks. Another advantage of the Power Port line is that it can last for years whereas most arm IV lines last only a few days.

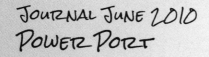

JOURNAL JUNE 2010
POWER PORT

In spite of waking up nauseated that morning I made it through surgery ok. Fortunately, they put me "out" for the procedure with general anesthesia. I woke up after with a fair amount of pain and worse nausea. But they gave me medication which resolved most of it. Sadly, the next day I was even sorer, still nauseated, and generally felt lousy. But the good news (sort of) was that I could finally begin my Lovenox (anticoagulant) injections.

Anticoagulant Therapy

Anticoagulants are usually called "blood thinners" by patients. This is technically not correct, but I rarely corrected my patients unless they wanted to know how it worked. These medications don't actually thin the blood. Instead they act on one or more clotting factors in the blood which results in slowing down the usual clotting time. The longer it takes for blood to form a clot, the more a person will bleed if injured so people who take them must follow certain precautions. In spite of the risk, anticoagulants may be appropriate for people with a DVT, a PE, heart attack, or other clot-related problems. This medication prevents further clot formation while the initial troublesome clot is slowly dissolved.

Journal June 2010
Injecting Myself

My doctor prescribed enxaparin (Lovenox) for my DVT in the form of a shot that I need to give myself daily. It goes into the fatty tissue of my abdomen. Fortunately, I have plenty of that in spite of some weight loss. I've given subcutaneous (SubQ) injections to my patients thousands of times over the years. But I discovered an interesting obstacle to giving myself an injection. It's called the pain reflex. It's that natural primal self-protective reflex we all have to pull our hand away from painful stimuli (like a hot stove). We don't consciously think about it. We just do it. It is an interesting reflex that bypasses the brain and is mediated at the spinal cord. So I used my expert dart-like injection technique to insert the needle into my tummy only to find myself immediately holding the syringe once again in front of me. Apparently my brain managed to insert the needle but my spinal cord immediately said "not so fast" and made my arm yank it back out. It was rather bizarre and unexpected. Matter over mind? Something like that. So I took a deep breath and assured myself that I WAS in control of my body and COULD do this. What followed was a total repeat of my first attempt. So there I was with two pokes in my belly, medication still in the syringe, a contaminated needle (nurse brain talking there) and feeling really stupid. I've given shots for 21 years. I've taught students to give shots for the past 17 years—and yet when it was crunch time I couldn't manage to give myself a shot? Good grief!

Not willing to admit defeat I took another deep slow breath, changed my strategy and did what I had always told my students NOT to do. I inserted the needle very slowly and intentionally so that my brain could remain in control the entire time. It hurt more but this time I was successful in keeping the needle inserted until I successfully depressed the plunger. If I had been grading myself as a student I would have failed because of the two failed attempts. But I decided to cut myself some slack under the circumstances. I managed to get the job done. But the next day I wimped out and let my daughter administer my shot.

Mind-Body Connection

I'd like to think that I am such an emotionally healthy person that I will cope effectively with my illness right up to the end. But this probably isn't true. The truth I've noticed is that it is so much easier to feel positive emotionally when I feel good physically. When I feel physically lousy, I notice, my attitude goes down the toilet. The radiation has done a number on my GI system and those related symptoms have worsened. Medication helps a little but only a little. Some days I want to crawl under my blankets and never come out. These are obviously the times I start whining. I want to stay strong and seek the learning and growth to be found during the hard times, but I need God's help. It's just too hard to do alone.

Chemotherapy

I've known a number of people who seemed to sail through chemotherapy. Of course that might not be how they would describe it. But I do know that they were able to keep working. Two different friends of mine had their chemo every Friday so they could recover over the weekend and be back to work on Monday; every week. How did they do it? How do any of them do it? Are they super human or am I just a complete wimp?

I felt a bit scared the first day in the infusion room. Fortunately, God answered another prayer and a friend that I used to work with at the hospital was there. She had many years of experience as an oncology nurse and I greatly admired her. I felt so relieved when she came for me in the waiting room. She was going to be my nurse for the day.

She began with the infusion of medications that were supposed to minimize nausea and then she infused the actual chemotherapy. It was a breeze. I remember thinking, "Well this was certainly easier than I expected. I don't know what all the fuss is about." My daughter and mother, who had come along for moral support, even took me to lunch afterwards and I was able to eat. I never expected that.

However, the nausea hit shortly after we got home. In my memory it's as if someone slowly turned down the dimmer switch. I recall just wanting to sleep until it passed. Unfortunately, it lasted for more than a week. Somewhere in the process is when I remember hearing my brother say "Promise me you won't give up." I may have replied but I don't recall. I was trapped in a dark pit of persistent nausea and just wanted to sleep.

Journal July 2010
Dehydration and Weight Loss

I realized after becoming extremely dehydrated last week that for some reason I don't have a good ability to identify dehydration in myself though I do a good job of identifying it in others (heck, I teach about this stuff in my Fluid and Electrolytes unit). Yet I got so out of balance. All I could tell at the time was that I felt super awful. I've been weighing myself every day to keep better track. How many times over my life have I tried to lose weight—usually with little success? Now I can't seem to stop losing.

Therapy Change

The plan had been to repeat the IV chemo every three weeks. I was quite worried about undergoing my second session since I still had not recovered from the first and I honestly questioned whether I could survive another round. So I was prepared for my next appointment with questions about whether the therapy might be modified to make it more tolerable. I wasn't ready to give up but really didn't want a repeat of the first go-round. As it turned out, we didn't even have that conversation. My oncologist immediately noted that I had tolerated the first treatment "very poorly" (no kidding!) and recommended a change. Tissue biopsy results had come back and indicated that my cancer cells have a certain "mutation" (sounds like a sci-fi movie) that makes me a good candidate for "targeted cell therapy." It would be in the form of a pill called Tarceva (erlotinib). It would not provide a cure but could extend my life by several years instead of the few months of my initial prognosis. The two most common side effects of Tarceva include diarrhea (which can be severe) and an acne-like rash that may be mild, moderate or severe. I prayed for the mild. My oncologist seemed more optimistic than in previous visits and stated that he felt he had something to offer that could make a significant difference. It does cause me to wonder why he recommended the chemo treatment in the first place, if he didn't think it would do much for me.

Tarceva is very expensive (around $5,000 per month) but thankfully my insurance covered most of it. I found myself feeling a bit guilty, though. Should I be the cause of so many healthcare dollars being spent on a medication that would not cure me? I felt a bit conflicted about this, yet I was not ready to lie down and die. So I took the Tarceva.

Swallowing Issues

I have issues with swallowing pills. I always have. As a child I used to hide my vitamins in the hollow metal leg of our dining room table. I recently told my mom. She laughed and shrugged. She thought I was getting all my vitamins when the table leg was getting them instead.

Despite my long history with swallowing issues, I didn't learn the underlying reason behind them until recently. Apparently a section of my esophagus is stenosed (narrowed) and doesn't work as well as the rest of it does. Consequently, pills or anything that's not chewed well have a tendency to get stuck there. I've had pills literally sit there for hours before they eventually dissolved or passed on down, so now I have to chew them instead of swallow them.

Some types of pills cannot be chewed. In this case I have found that I can usually get them down with food. I mention this because Tarceva cannot be cut, crushed, or chewed. I was supposed to swallow them whole, on an empty stomach. Well that's not happening. So I talked with a pharmacist who said I could get away with eating a couple of bites of food. That was a relief. Now to identify which food worked best.

JOURNAL JULY 2010
TARCEVA THERAPY

On day one I swallowed my first Tarceva pill with a couple of bites of bread and some water. It worked okay, but not great. On day three I tried covering the pill in some butter which worked better. After two weeks of experimenting with different foods I discovered that banana works the best. I only need a bite or two. It's got enough substance to carry the pill down to my stomach, and enough moisture to keep it from getting stuck. In the hospital and nursing homes we use pudding or apple sauce. Sometimes it works and sometimes it doesn't. I like the banana. Roxy (my dog) likes it too. Bananas are one of her favorite treats. Since I don't need more than a couple of bites, we share it (the banana, not the Tarceva).

Tarceva Therapy

My first few months on Tarceva went reasonably well, all things considered. I did develop the facial rash which was very tender but I was fortunate and only developed the mild version. I cannot imagine having the severe form. After several weeks it went away, which I did not expect but am so grateful for. The GI distress and diarrhea, which had already begun as a side effect of radiation, progressively worsened until I had been on Tarceva for at least a month. If I could do it all over again I would choose three weeks of radiation instead of two. I think spreading it out a bit might have been gentler on my GI system. Of course the chemo probably had an impact too. Fortunately, by the end of August it began to slowly improve. I also began to slowly regain my appetite and stopped losing weight.

The month of September included a variety of journal entries in which I whined (a lot) about fatigue, a nine-day headache, eye pain, visual changes, other aches and pains, two upper respiratory infections, and symptoms of a possible infection (fever, chills, etc.).

October was another month full of so many aches and pains that I again decided to summarize them. My vision slowly worsened, especially in my right eye. I felt as though I was looking through a milky haze or film. I also had a headache, a stiff, sore neck that made turning my head difficult. My eyes felt quite sore, hurt to move, and were tender to touch. I debated about whether to call my doctor, but complaining about every little thing was making me feel like a hypochondriac. Of course I also complained frequently of fatigue. All I wanted to do was sleep. And when I wasn't sleeping I wished I was.

I was doing okay from a spiritual/emotional standpoint. I had my moments, especially if I felt poor physically, when I want to curl up and hide under a blanket (and sometimes I did). But I keep asking God to remind me of the many things I have to be grateful for and there are always so many things. It helps me keep my focus.

My blood tests were okay, except some anemia which is no surprise for a cancer patient. It also explained some of my ongoing fatigue. The scans indicated no new cancer spots anywhere, the sacral lesion was unchanged, and the lung tumor had shrunk significantly. My doctor said this was the best we could have hoped for based on what they've seen with Tarceva. So to be clear, I was not cured, but this definitely indicated the medication was doing its job and I was getting more time and better quality for much of that time. "Thank you Lord." I still struggled with eating much of the time. I wasn't losing weight anymore which was good, but I worked to get enough calories in. I think I was maintaining my weight due to my ice cream "therapy." My kids kept urging me to try the medical marijuana pills so I finally asked my oncologist about them. He gave me a prescription so I could try it out.

JOURNAL NOVEMBER 2010 MARINOL

I tried taking Marinol. It left me feeling rather worthless all day (more than usual) and made me even more sleepy than usual. I couldn't hold a train of thought for two seconds (or so it seemed), I felt pretty fuzzy-headed and watching TV was quite interesting. I kept seeing it in a sort of 3-D that I can't quite describe. Bizarre. I'm not so sure it helped my appetite which was the whole point. And I don't like how I lost my afternoon, so doubt I'll take it again.

Consultations

My eye pain and visual changes finally prompted me to make an eye appointment. I wondered if it would be a waste of time but it revealed some interesting findings. The eye doctor didn't think any of it was related to my cancer or the Tarceva. However, the rheumatologist I saw shortly thereafter disagreed and was quite sure it was caused by the Tarceva. It would be nice if they could all agree. Anyway my eye doctor said I was having an episode of acute (closed) angle glaucoma when I had the recent severe headache and eye pain. He also diagnosed me with iritis (inflammation of the iris, probably related to the glaucoma). Further, he said there was evidence that my right iris was "stuck" (probably during the acute glaucoma) and when it finally came "unstuck" it left a ring of pigment in my right eye which is responsible for much of my vision symptoms. Apparently this is permanent. He also said that I had some cataract development in progress, especially in the right eye. And as if that weren't all enough, I also had inflammatory nodules around the right iris (quite a bit) and in the left eye (less). The only good news was that I guess I'm not a hypochondriac and the anti-inflammatory eye drops he prescribed resolved most of my eye problems.

It seems that my life is not to follow a smooth course any more (health-wise). The weird thing is that nothing he said really bothered me. I told Nicole I think it's because I've already heard the worst news you can hear from a doctor . . . so by comparison nothing else really seems so bad. In fact, I found myself thinking "Well I probably won't live long enough for this to become a real problem."

Teaching

Below the neck I've been feeling okay (all things considered). I wanted to continue to work if I could so I was assigned the Monday night Medical Terminology class. It is one of the easiest since I've taught it for so many years and, of course, literally wrote the book. I've also attended a few meetings and helped a bit in the nursing lab. But that's all. My energy level was very low—maybe thirty percent of what it was in the past—and what energy I had got used up quickly, but I was finally adapting to that and was getting better at pacing myself. Now and then I had a day where I felt totally wiped out and had no real explanation, but it didn't happen quite as often as it used to. I did have some pain in my sacrum which had worsened a bit. But fortunately it is managed pretty well with medication. I was so grateful that I'd had no pulmonary symptoms thus far and I prayed this continued.

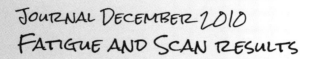

Journal December 2010
Fatigue and Scan Results

My fatigue continues on as annoying as ever. Yesterday I met with my oncologist who said my scans looked "great," meaning they were essentially unchanged from three months ago. He doesn't think my fatigue is caused by the cancer, but that it might be the Tarceva. I think it's both. They drew blood to monitor my anemia which continues to be a problem. But I've seen worse in other cancer patients.

Naturopath Consult

I believe that natural measures can be helpful in certain situations so I went to a naturopathic physician to learn what I might do to boost my body's healing powers. She was very nice and seemed knowledgeable. She was generous with her time, spending a good two hours with me. However, it turned out that my oncologist advised against most of the measures she recommended. Oddly, although a diet high in anti-oxidants is generally a good thing and is believed to help prevent cancer—studies have apparently shown that people who already have cancer actually die sooner when they go on such diets. The reason is unclear but current thought is that it interferes with the cancer treatment or the body's own immune defenses. Consequently, I decided to eat and drink whatever sounds good, take my regular vitamins, and follow my oncologist's advice.

Over the months I've received so many suggestions about how to treat my cancer and my mother has also been the benefactor of information from well-meaning relatives. So I needed to find a way to explain to her why I wasn't jumping on all the various bandwagons that roll by. In doing so I came up with a sports analogy, which is sort of funny given that neither of us is a big sports fan. But it seemed to work for her because she completely understood and never questioned me about it again. It also seemed to help her know how to respond to the well-meaning friends and relatives who kept giving her advice to pass along to me.

JOURNAL FEBRUARY 2011
THE "COACH" THEORY

I told my mother that if I let myself, I could go nuts bouncing from one "expert" to another, trying the dozens of purported miracle cures out there. In the process it would likely interfere with my medication and treatment plan, ruin my quality of life, and use up all my money. I think of athletes who may have numerous coaches and a stand full of armchair quarterbacks all giving conflicting advice (all with good intentions). If they try to follow everyone's advice they will drive themselves nuts and surely won't perform well. The better option is to identify the head coach and follow his or her plan. So I decided that my oncologist is my head coach. We have a collaborative relationship and so far, he listens to me. I must put a certain degree of trust in his expertise. So for now, I choose to follow his advice. If at any point in the future, I dislike where he's taking me, then I will get a second opinion or change coaches. But for now it's him. This makes my life simpler and less stressful.

Energy, or Lack Thereof

My energy level continued to fluctuate between low and absurdly low although I noticed a slight improvement which might have been a delayed response to reducing my Tarceva dosage several months earlier. I started on the full adult dose of 150mg per day and had reduced it to 100mg instead. The goal was to find the lowest dose that would still achieve the same results in hopes of reducing side effects, which in my case, was mostly the profound, chronic fatigue.

I didn't have the necessary energy to return to work other than the few things I was currently doing but was grateful to feel well enough to occasionally write, do a load of laundry, or a bit of light housework. I couldn't do much at any given time or even within the same day so I was learning to pace myself and prioritize how I use my energy. Family and friends usually came first.

JOURNAL MAY 2011
FATIGUE

The fatigue feels so pervasive and overwhelming I must constantly summon energy just to fight it off. I get so very tired of feeling so tired. What little energy I have is quickly depleted and resting only helps a little. I so miss that feeling of waking up refreshed after a good night's sleep. I've nearly forgotten what it feels like. Even when I sleep well, all I want to do after I get up is take a nap. So I usually just sit in my recliner and stare at the wall until I either go back to bed or summon the energy to actually do something. This is probably the one thing that most diminishes my quality of life. If I'm fighting any sort of "battle" here it's not with the cancer itself but rather with the fatigue. Sometimes I wonder, when I die, if it will just be a matter of finally giving in to the fatigue and drifting away. That doesn't seem like such a bad thing . . . when it's time. Not that I'm ready now, but feeling this way makes me wonder.

Pain

My pain issues were very slowly worsening. Sorting it out was tricky. There was the painful metastatic lesion (cancerous spot) on my left sacrum (very low back/buttocks). This is bone pain which is well known for being severe and challenging to treat. I also felt worsening pain and tenderness in my joints; especially my knees and shoulders. This is a known side effect of Tarceva. However, it could also have been the inevitable joint pain caused by arthritis associated with aging. Occasionally I also felt a deep radiating pain in my left shoulder and arm which is also a known symptom among lung cancer patients.

JOURNAL JULY 2011
PAIN

I'm puzzled that my oncologist seems not to have heard of any of the symptoms described above. When I describe them he just looks at me and says "Huh" like it's the first time he's ever heard such a thing. So it makes me wonder if he is trying to downplay my symptoms so he can ignore them. Or is he really ignorant about all of this? Having a physician who shrugs off my complaints is troublesome. Having a physician who is ignorant about the symptoms of lung cancer and side effects of a major form of treatment is worse. He just fixates on the two issues of facial rash and diarrhea and refuses to acknowledge any others. And he asks me about them on every single visit even though I have repeatedly told him that they have resolved. Most annoying. I'm beginning to feel like I know more about Tarceva than he does.

From Workaholic to Couch Potato

Before my diagnosis, I was a workaholic. Because there was always so much to do, I was obsessed with being productive and excelled at multitasking. I hated to ever "waste" time. It all began years ago when I entered nursing school and continued right on through graduate school and my various nursing jobs. I was also a single mom so there was never a shortage of things on my "To Do" list. It became a lifestyle and I would have been bored to tears and incredibly restless if I just sat around home all day as I do now. Given this, one might expect that I would hate the slow pace of my life these days. But I don't. Having less energy changes things. I find that I still feel "busy" but it is a different sort of busyness. Whereas in the past I was limited by time, I now feel limited by inadequate energy. My body requires me to rest often and pace myself, so somehow it works out that I'm not left feeling bored at all.

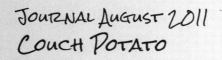

JOURNAL AUGUST 2011
COUCH POTATO

Since I generally feel least well in the mornings I've fallen into a pattern of staying awake fairly late and then sleeping in. I spend most of my day on my laptop, cuddling my puppy (who has WAY more energy than I do), reading, watching TV, or napping. I don't get too much done at any given time. My favorite place to rest is a new "mini" recliner in the corner of my bedroom. It's just the right size for my short body and Roxy likes the footrest because it provides a good place to nap.

Anorexia

Most non-medical people confuse anorexia, loss of appetite, with anorexia nervosa, the eating disorder where a person intentionally starves herself. The two types are very different. Anorexia nervosa is a psychiatric disorder with physical manifestations. Plain anorexia is simply the loss of appetite from any number of physical causes. Examples include medication side effects, pregnancy, and various illnesses.

JOURNAL OCTOBER 2011
ANOREXIA

Anorexia associated with cancer reminds me a little of when I was pregnant, but in that case it was time limited and there was a baby to look forward to. With cancer the emotional dimension is more challenging. There is no baby and I can never be sure if or when I will feel better.

When working with cancer patients I recall thinking they ought to be able to reason things through intellectually and know that although they don't feel like eating, they should force themselves to. Common sense dictates that we need nutrition and a certain number of calories to heal and feel better. It's obvious, or so I thought. I am now realizing that I underestimated how difficult it really is.

Like most Americans, I've spent most of my life in love with food. I especially loved Italian and most types of Asian foods. I also had a special fondness for good ole American comfort foods with sauces and gravies as well as rich desserts like cheesecake, ice cream, pies, and pastries. In my culture most activities revolve around food. This includes social and family gatherings as well as celebrations of all sorts from weddings to funerals and everything in between. Consequently, like most Americans, when I look in the mirror I think I'd look better if I were a bit thinner and I've struggled to lose the same ten to twenty pounds for most of my adult life.

This all suddenly changed when I developed serious anorexia last summer after my initial round of IV chemotherapy. Not only did I lose the desire to eat, but the look, smell or thought of food was nauseating. The fact that social activities are so closely tied to food became its own challenge. I rarely felt like leaving the house, but didn't want to miss opportunities to be with family and friends. I no longer took such opportunities for granted and treasured my time with loved ones.

Gatherings in my home or the home of a friend were most comfortable since I could seek the comfort of a recliner or sofa when needed. Eating in restaurants was more challenging. I had to try to make myself presentable for the public, had a limited choice of seating, and was surrounded by a wider range of sights and smells than usual. It was always a struggle to identify anything on the menu that seemed even remotely appealing. Once my food arrived I'd usually only manage a few bites before giving up. Eventually I learned to not order at all. Instead, my friends and family shared very tiny portions of some of their meals with me. It was much more practical, saved money, and spared me the pressure and guilt of leaving a full plate behind.

After several months the initial anorexia improved

somewhat, but lately has worsened again. I'm hoping it's a passing phase. Most days I have zero appetite and am slightly nauseated—just enough that the thought of food makes it worse. Sometimes I can force myself to eat something anyway. But the problem with eating is that we need to keep doing it. It's not like a dose of medication that I can take once or twice and be done with it. The issue just never goes away. Day after day I'm supposed to keep eating. It becomes an exhausting chore that never gets any easier.

Nails and Skin

When people ask me about treatment side effects I usually assume they want the abbreviated, sanitized answer. In this case, I usually respond with something like, "There are lots of little things, but mostly I just feel tired all the time." Most of the time, they are satisfied with this answer which indicates my assumption was correct. However, if they want an honest, detailed answer, my response becomes much longer.

Tarceva impacts the skin and all skin-related structures. During the first year I struggled with infections around the toenails on my big toes, which was something I'd never encountered before. It began as mild tenderness and quickly evolved into a nasty case of ingrown toenails. Both toes were affected and became so painful that I could only wear sandals, regardless of the weather, so as to eliminate any pressure on them. I began daily soaks which helped some, but only temporarily. It became a chronic issue that impacted my quality of life. So after procrastinating way too long, I finally made an appointment with a podiatrist (foot doctor). He performed a procedure in which he numbed both toes and removed the outer nail edges of each toe. Aftercare involved frequent soaking and dressing changes. Fortunately, they healed quickly and have not been a problem since.

My finger and toenails are weaker than before and split and break much more easily. My skin has also changed, becoming drier and coarser with lots of "age" spots. This might have been upsetting to me in the past, but now I take it all in stride. I feel more aware than ever that I am not my body. It is simply a vessel in which I temporarily reside and one day I will leave it behind.

Trigger Thumb

Then there's my thumbs. Over the past six to eight months I've developed trigger thumb, first on the right, then a few months later, on the left. I'm not sure if this had anything to do with the Tarceva. But given how it affects joints, it seems a possibility.

First I noticed the distal (nearest to the end) thumb joint sticking in place. With more force I could get it to bend and noted an unpainful popping sensation. It was mild at first but became more pronounced over time. Then pain and tenderness developed in all thumb joints, especially the middle one. I could also feel a hard bump at the thumb's base which became more pronounced over time. When I began dropping things due to pain and weakness I decided it was time to see the doctor. I was fortunate enough to see an orthopedic doctor who specializes in hand disorders. He confirmed the diagnosis and said I had two options. A corticosteroid injection would provide temporary relief. Surgery would provide a permanent fix. He said it rarely improves on its own so I should probably schedule surgery. But being a good procrastinator and not currently dependent on my hands or fingers for work, I decided to use the wait-and-see approach. I'm not eager to undergo any procedures or surgeries I don't really need. At this time, they both seem to have improved somewhat so I'm going to give it more time.

Body Hair

Speaking of weird side effects there are a number of others I've failed to mention before now. My leg hair growth has slowed down which is a nice perk. My underarm hair has nearly disappeared and my eyebrow hair became darker, coarser, and longer. My eyelashes have changed shape so none of them go in the same direction anymore. It's like they've gone wild. Some curl backwards and poke my eyeball (and must be plucked out), others grow in a corkscrew pattern and a few have actually straightened so they stick straight out. Many have also fallen out leaving bare spots. Mascara only accentuates all the weirdness so I've given up wearing any.

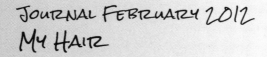

JOURNAL FEBRUARY 2012
MY HAIR

The hair on my head has developed an absurdly strong, weird, asymmetrical growth pattern. On my left side it insists on laying straight forward against my scalp. On my right it has developed a strange part from front to back. Hair above the part grows straight up and hair below grows downward. All of it has also become coarser than usual. There is no styling it. Applying super-hold gel has no lasting effect. After a few minutes the hair bounces back and goes where it wants. So I had my daughter cut it all off with electric clippers. It's a relief to not have to bother with it anymore. The only real downside is I must now protect my head from the summer heat and winter cold. So although I never considered myself a hat person in the past, I now have a growing hat collection. People who notice my super short hair sometimes assume that I lost it through chemo and make well-meaning comments about how nicely it is "growing back." Occasionally I tell them the truth which is that I never lost it, but most of the time I just say "thanks" and leave it at that. I had been told I would lose all my hair with that first chemo treatment. It thinned a bit in front and that was it. My sweet middle son was almost disappointed because he had planned on shaving his head in support. I told him I appreciated the thought but was glad he didn't need to.

Changing Doctors

Although my oncologist seems to be a nice man, over time, I found myself feeling less than satisfied with his care. It was small things at first but over time they began to add up. Each visit began the same. "Are you having any problem with diarrhea or facial rash?" he'd say as he looked more closely at my face. Each time I gave the exact same response: "Only some mild problems in the first few months, nothing since." But what went through my mind at the time was, "Do you realize you ask me the very same question every time? Don't you take notes? I feel like you run on autopilot and haven't given my individual case any thought since the first two months." As time went by I felt less and less like he was listening to me. He began shrugging off most of my comments, by acting like he'd never heard such a thing before. While the Tarceva is clearly the cause of my fatigue he kept blaming the pain medication. This might be true in situations where opioids are taken short term for acute pain. However, when they are taken regularly, over time, the side effects of sedation, respiratory depression, and fatigue disappear. This means they should no longer be an issue of concern except in situations where the dosage is suddenly and significantly increased (something we never did). My oncologist should have known this. But as time went by he kept beating this drum and seemed fixated on reducing or eliminating my pain medication (see chapter 12). On some visits he also blamed my fatigue on the Tarceva (likely correct). Yet at other times he responded as if he'd never heard of it before. Although I believed him to be a well-intentioned man, this all left me feeling as though he wasn't doing his homework and had lost interest in my case. So after a great deal of thought, deliberation, and a conversation with my primary care doctor, I changed oncologists.

Nearly Three Years Later . . .

For the next three years I continued on the Tarceva with good results (meaning no significant changes in my scans). I was even able to further reduce the dosage to 75mg per day. My energy level improved only slightly but I did regain my appetite and also regained the lost weight. In fact, I managed to gain even more weight which I'm not too thrilled about. However, having seen how quickly it falls off when I'm ill, I decided to just try to keep it steady. I'm not attempting to lose it but I certainly don't want to gain any more either. Side effects already described continued on but were minimal until Thanksgiving, 2014.

Intolerable Side Effects

I missed Thanksgiving 2014. Shortly before then, I began having episodes of severe GI distress. It began with a weird sort of bloating unlike any I've ever had followed by increased belching (burping), diarrhea, and gas. It hit after dinner in the early evening and kept me awake much of the night. I felt somewhat better by morning. But that evening it recurred and the pattern repeated itself. Thinking it was something I had eaten, I became very cautious about my diet, but I found that made no difference. Sadly, this all occurred over Thanksgiving so instead of spending the day with my family, I spent the day in bed (between toilet trips). In addition to feeling physically ill, I also felt emotionally down that day as I pictured the rest of my family gathered together at my son's house and knew I was missing out. It made me wonder if this were a sign of what the future held in store. Would I find myself more frequently feeling ill and be stuck in bed for Christmas, New Year's, and other special days to come? I later learned that it was an especially difficult and painful day for my son, Brian, who found himself having similar thoughts as well as wondering if we'd already spent our last Thanksgiving together.

Recalling that diarrhea is one of the major side effects of Tarceva I called my doctor who instructed me to take a two week Tarceva "holiday" (time off the medication) which was fine by me. The GI problems immediately resolved and I resumed the Tarceva as before. I felt fine for about two weeks and then the same pattern repeated itself, more severe than before. Upon my doctor's instructions I took a second Tarceva holiday and once again the symptoms resolved.

The third time around was much worse than before. Severe stomach cramps kept me awake all night, along with nausea and severe diarrhea. By morning I was dehydrated (in spite of drinking fluids) and had no energy. So I went to the clinic where I received IV fluids, and anti-diarrhea and antinausea medication. My symptoms improved significantly and I was able to return home. This time the stomach pain, tenderness, and occasional cramping continued for several more days before it finally resolved. By this point the pattern was very clear and I was convinced that Tarceva was the cause. My oncologist wanted me to resume the Tarceva at a reduced dose but given the progressive severity of my symptoms I wasn't ready. So we agreed I could remain off the Tarceva until the next scheduled scans.

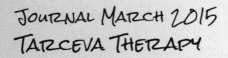

JOURNAL MARCH 2015
TARCEVA THERAPY

I think I'm done with the Tarceva. My scans looked good so my oncologist recommended I remain off as long as I can to let my gut have lots of healing time. That's fine with me. I really cannot complain. Many people don't tolerate Tarceva at all and it's given me more than four and a half years. God does answer prayer. I asked for more time. He has given it to me and I am grateful.

Cancer has a powerful impact on all who have it, regardless of type. This is especially true for those with stages 3 and 4. The gritty and sometimes scary side to this disease involves the treatments, procedures, side effects, and complications. Despite whatever support system patients may have, they often feel like they face these things alone.

Chapter 2 Notes

1. Maggie Smith, "Brainy Quotes," Maggie Smith Quotes, November 2, 2015. http://www.brainyquote.com/quotes/authors/m/maggie_smith.html

Chapter 3:
Nurse and Educator

When I think about all the patients and their loved ones that I have worked with over the years, I know most of them don't remember me nor I them, but I do know that I gave a little piece of myself to each of them and they to me and those threads make up the beautiful tapestry in my mind that is my career in nursing.[1]

When my kids were small I was a full-time mother and homemaker and I loved it. Yet I also knew that I wanted a career but was unsure what it would be. I only knew that I wanted and needed to feel that I was somehow making a difference in the world. The funny thing was that I ended up doing the very things I'd said I would never do. At different times in my earlier life I had said that I would never be a nurse and I would never be a teacher. Yet I ended up doing both and loved it. So what changed? It was my understanding of what nurses and teachers do.

My concept of nursing, like that of most people, was totally wrong. I thought it was all bedpans, baths and pills, and doing what the doctor told me without thinking for myself. I wanted to do something more interesting and mentally challenging than cleaning bums and following someone else's orders. I wanted a career that allowed me some autonomy and creativity to do things in my own way. I eventually learned that nursing is a great career path that allows for exactly these things. And so is teaching. But what triggered my change of heart?

The day I met and spoke with members of a Heartflight medical team at a summer conference, I realized that nursing was so much more than I had thought.[2] I was blown away by their transport team which was comprised largely of nurses. They did interesting, challenging, exciting things. They rescued people and saved lives. They flew all over the Pacific Northwest treating and transporting the sickest of the sick. People so ill or injured that they were unlikely to survive unless they got to a level one trauma center during the Golden Hour (first sixty minutes after injury). This experience was an eye-opener for me and was so inspiring that I drove to the local community college the very next day and spoke to the director of the nursing program. From that day on, my path was clear. I would become a nurse. I would save and impact lives. I would make a difference.

Becoming a Nurse

Though I had already earned a four-year degree in Sociology I had always avoided science and math courses. This partly stemmed from the fact that the only time I attempted a chemistry class, I earned a D. I believe it was the only D of my college career and it was embarrassing. I was terrified at the idea of ever stepping into a chemistry class again.

I had to face my fears ten years later when I decided I wanted to be a nurse. I couldn't let this one science class stand as an obstacle between me and my chosen profession, so I put on my big girl panties (along with the rest of my clothes) and walked into that classroom. To my surprise and relief, I found it quite interesting. I loved the class and earned an A. It's amazing what can happen when one puts forth the required energy to attend class and study.

In addition to the chemistry course I needed to take several other prerequisite classes before I could enter the nursing program. Therefore, it took me three years to earn a two-year degree as a registered nurse. The classes were much more difficult than anything I had taken at the university but I loved them all, except maybe the math. I never learned to like it but I did learn that I could do it. I was especially fascinated to learn how the human body works and most of the sciences I'd avoided in my earlier education, were now my favorites.

Like other nursing students I spent part of my week in the classroom and part of it in the clinical setting. There I selected patients to learn about and care for. It was challenging and scary and wonderful all at the same time. Fortunately, I discovered I am a people person so with time and practice it became fairly easy to meet new people and establish rapport within a short time frame. My approach, which combined honest sincerity with subtle humor seemed to put most of them quickly at ease. I found it deeply rewarding to help them feel better, emotionally and physically. Though I was unsure what area I would specialize in, I knew I was on the right path and was meant to be a nurse.

Family Sacrifice

Being a full time student and a single parent of three wasn't easy. Both aspects of my life were very demanding and it seemed I always felt guilty regardless of how I allotted my time. When I was busy studying, I feared I was neglecting my kids. When I spent time with my kids, I feared I was neglecting my studies. I suspect most working mothers can relate to this. We want to believe we can "have it all," but it always comes at a price. I think this is probably when my mantras about being productive and not wasting time began. It felt like there just weren't enough hours in the day. I tried to utilize every minute, so it wasn't unusual to see me flipping through flash cards or reading an assignment while sitting in the orthodontist's waiting room or watching my kids play soccer.

I tried to make myself feel better by choosing to believe that my studies were an investment in my family's future. In those days, women were often still made to feel guilty if they "abandoned" their families for a career. But I knew it was important to be a strong role model for my children; something I hadn't done so well in their earliest years. I wanted them, especially my daughter, to know that it's okay for women (and moms) to have careers so they can do meaningful work, earn money, and take care of their families. I hoped, eventually, they would realize that our sacrifice was worth it, and they might one day even be proud of me. I wanted to believe all of this and hoped I wasn't just kidding myself. There were many days along the way that were difficult. Times when they wanted me to play but I had to study for an exam. Times when they needed to stay with other family or a sitter while I went to class or clinical. I knew I was not the only one making sacrifices. But ultimately it was all worth it.

One day, a couple of years into the process, I overheard my kids bragging to the neighbor kids as they played in the back yard. One of them said "Our mom is going to college to be a nurse. She is going to save people's lives." I remained out of sight as tears of relief ran down my face. My kids were proud of me. I felt so relieved and grateful and also proud of my children for recognizing that what we were working together to build was ultimately worthwhile. A short time later they attended my pinning ceremony at the college where they could see how I was recognized for my accomplishment. Five years later they attended another graduation at the university where they saw me earn my master's degree. They were proud. And they were grateful it was over. So was I.

I know I've made many mistakes as a mother and I do have a few regrets. However, my children have turned into awesome adults whom I love having in my life. They are good, honest, hardworking people. So I choose to believe that their father and I did more things right than wrong. And by the way, did I mention that my daughter became a nurse too? It wasn't my idea. It was hers. And she isn't just a nurse. She is an excellent nurse; probably better than I ever was.

A Clinical Challenge

In addition to personal challenges at home, there were professional ones as well. In fact, one day I encountered a challenge I couldn't overcome and for a brief time, found myself questioning my chosen career path. I was on an orthopedic rotation where most patients were recovering from broken bones or joint replacement surgery. It was pretty straight forward; there were very few medications and nearly all patients were expected to get better and return home.

I arrived early on Friday morning prepared to care for the patient I had selected, studied, and cared for the previous day. But when I entered her room I was shocked to find her gone. I learned from the charge nurse that she had been discharged the evening before, earlier than expected. I was happy for her but disheartened that I wouldn't be able to be her nurse for a second day. I approached my clinical instructor regarding my patient-less status, and she assigned me a new patient.

Mr. Henry had been admitted during the night with a complex ankle fracture that had required surgery. He had made it through the post-op phase and was now resting in his bed, sleepy but oriented and mostly comfortable. He was a friendly fellow who welcomed the extra TLC a student could provide although in reality his main problem of post-operative pain was being well controlled with his PCA pump. This pump allowed him to dose himself with pain medication when his pain increased and kept him fairly comfortable. Because he was a last minute assignment, and the physician had the chart, I decided to go ahead and get acquainted and perform the physical assessment. At this point the only data I had on him was his name, age, and admitting diagnosis. This meant I was operating without having the historical data I was used to. I performed the exam and vital signs, then prepared to leave him with his breakfast, while I did my "homework." As I began to walk away he commented that he didn't know if his ankle would have time to heal before he died. This caught me by surprise and he responded to my questioning look by stating, "My cancer was quite advanced by the time they found it, so I don't have very long." I don't remember exactly what I said. I think I mumbled some form of condolences and said I'd be back to check on him after breakfast. What I recall clearly is exiting his room to the hallway as I tried to catch my breath, then leaning against the wall for support. I found myself overwhelmed with this new information. It had hit me like a large wave and took my breath away. My first thought was "I can't fix this! I can't fix this and I don't know how to help him! What do I do?" I suddenly felt completely powerless and terrified of walking back into his room.

I took a short break in the nurse's lounge to gather my thoughts. Then I got my hands on his chart and quickly read through his history. Sure enough. There it was. Stage IV lung cancer. Terminal. Life expectancy at the time of the diagnosis was only six months. That was nearly five months ago. He was going to die soon and there was nothing I could do about it.

I did my best to regroup and spent the rest of my shift providing the best nursing care and TLC I could. But for the next week I found myself reeling from the situation. I wanted to be a nurse. I wanted to help people. But the realization that some patients would die regardless of my intentions or good care, was almost more than I could bear. For the first time in nearly two years I found myself questioning my decision to become a nurse.

It was as if God spoke to the classroom instructor about my dilemma. The next week as we all busily took notes during the lecture, she paused and talked for a few minutes about dying patients. I'm sure she said a number of valuable things, but what I remember, what I needed to hear that day was this: "You cannot fix everything and you cannot fix everyone. That is not your job. Your job is to provide the best nursing care you can, and let God take care of the rest." As I pondered this I felt a huge weight lift from my shoulders. I realized I had been trying to take on a responsibility that wasn't mine. I wasn't God. I'm still not. My job then and now is simply to handle what is laid before me, and let Him take care of the rest.

Novice Nurse

Upon graduation in 1989, I was hired to work in the most challenging area I knew of, the Medical/Oncology unit of the same hospital where I'd spent most of my clinical rotations. As a student I'd been overwhelmed by the complexity of patients on that unit. Yet I believed I was up for the challenge; I felt it would prepare me to go anywhere from there. And it was true.

I worked twelve-hour nights for the next two and a half years providing care for the sickest and most complicated patients outside of the critical care area. Adult, mostly elderly patients with three to five pages of medications, lengthy lists of diagnoses and complex histories were the norm. Typical patient diagnoses included liver diseases like hepatitis and cirrhosis, bowel diseases like Crohn's disease, diverticulitis, bowel obstructions, and gastrointestinal bleeds. Roughly a third of the patients also had diabetes and many suffered from non-healing infections requiring amputations. Some had pancreatitis, an inflammation of the pancreas. Many had lung disease, the most common being chronic obstructive pulmonary disease (COPD). There were infections of all sorts including those resistant to antibiotics. Among the most behaviorally challenging patients were those with dementia, those with meningitis (which often caused confusion and agitation), and those who had attempted suicide. Part of the unit was reserved for cancer patients and though I didn't specialize as an oncology (cancer) nurse I still cared for many patients with all types of cancer. This was also where I cared for my first patient with AIDs.

As a student in the late eighties I recall that AIDs was the hot topic of the day and was considered a death sentence for any who contracted it. Life expectancy was something like twelve to eighteen months. I recall many philosophical and ethical conversations among classmates in which we naïvely believed we could choose whom we would and wouldn't care for. Yet, later as a graduate nurse when assigned my first known AIDs patient, I didn't think twice about it. He was ill and he needed a nurse. I became a nurse to help people, so I didn't flinch when I saw him on my patient list. I took care of him for three nights in a row and at least two of those nights were unusually calm which allowed me the luxury of spending extra time with him. I became acquainted with him as a person rather than a statistic. He was an attractive man in his late thirties who believed he'd contracted AIDs through casual, heterosexual sex. He was kind, thoughtful, intelligent, and deeply introspective. He was frightened he might die, and very much wanted to live. He'd been admitted with a type of pneumonia common in people with AIDs. His last night with me he developed a cough, but I didn't think he looked or acted like someone in danger of dying soon. When I returned from several days off I learned he'd been transferred to critical care. He died two weeks later. I felt sad and concerned I might have missed some clue regarding the gravity of his condition. I wondered, if I'd noticed some clue and transferred him sooner might he have lived longer? It haunted me for months, but as I thought it all over I realized that in my mind and heart he had transformed from a statistic into a real person I cared about. This made it more difficult to acknowledge he was far more ill than I had wanted to admit. I finally accepted that I gave him the best care possible under the circumstances and managed to let it go. The "if onlys" can drive you nuts in this profession. I wrestled with them many times but eventually accepted that all I could do was my very best given my knowledge and resources at the time. I couldn't see into the future. I could only handle what was in front of me.

The Medical/Oncology unit provided a fertile learning ground. Because our patients were not hooked up to high tech monitoring devices, I learned the value of developing good observation and physical assessment skills. Over time, I also learned to trust my nurse's judgment and gut instinct. I learned the importance of really looking at, and listening to, my patients. As I later often told my students, "Patients are experts on their own bodies so we must listen to them." I came to realize that good nurses become a sort of medical detective as they gather all the clues that manifest in the form of test results, vital signs, physical exam findings, medical history, medications, patient statements, physician notes, and so on.

The good nurse considers all pieces of the puzzle to gain an understanding of the whole patient picture. Good nurses not only respond appropriately to patients in crisis but, when possible, take proactive measures to prevent the crisis. Good nurses take their role as patient advocate seriously. This means they are willing to assertively communicate with doctors and other team members, regardless of the hour, to get patients whatever they need.

I did not immediately become a good nurse although I certainly wanted to. I recall wishing I could just wake up the next day with five years of nursing experience behind me. But like everyone else, I had to start at the beginning. It takes time, practice, mentoring from more experienced nurses, and the willingness to work hard and be teachable. Slowly, over much time, I became a good nurse.

Advanced Nurse

From the Medical/Oncology unit I transferred to critical care (also called the intensive care unit or ICU) where I worked four more years of twelve hour nights. It, too, was a rich learning environment and I enjoyed the challenges there. This is where most nurses who love the high-tech stuff end up. They, along with emergency nurses, are often called "adrenaline junkies" because they love the challenges posed by unstable, critically ill patients. In the ICU, patients often appear surrounded by a "jungle" of machines, pumps, tubes, drains, IV lines, and other paraphernalia. Each item serves an important purpose but the same environment that nurses find challenging and exciting is usually overwhelming and frightening for patients and families. Because of this, I made a point of explaining, in a simple manner, the purpose of each. For this they often voiced their appreciation.

Because the ICU (at that time) was essentially one huge open area with curtains that could be drawn between patients, I was able to observe my coworkers more closely than on other nursing units. In doing so, I noticed how their personal styles influenced the type of care they gave. In most cases it wasn't a matter of doing things right or wrong but it did translate into doing things differently. And in my opinion this difference sometimes had a huge impact on the patients and their loved ones.

In general, I noticed three nursing personality types. The first group was very rules-driven and often viewed the world in black and white, right and wrong. Give them one of those paint-by-number projects and they would likely produce beautiful pictures with everything painted perfectly and always according to directions. They would never, ever paint outside the lines. These type of people like to follow rules to the letter. Technically speaking they were usually excellent nurses because they paid close attention to details, were hard workers, and made sure that everything got done according to plan. They were often the ones referred to as adrenaline junkies. They also seemed to have a high need to be in control of their surroundings. Part of the reason they loved the ICU is that things can quickly go wrong and chaos always threatens to ensue. For them the challenge was to maintain control and keep chaos at bay. They thrived on controlling everything, including the patient, the immediate environment and to some degree, those around them. They were the ones that loved to enforce all rules including those pertaining to visitation. If the rules stated "family members only, a maximum of two at a time, for a maximum of ten minutes each hour" then that was it. They were the ones who might argue that the significant other didn't qualify for visitation because they weren't married. They also seemed to find other "conditions" that disallowed visitors more often than other nurses. For example, anytime they were administering patient care, or the patient, or his/her neighbor were undergoing a procedure, and certainly whenever there was an emergency anywhere within the ICU. This could all add up to endless hours in which loved ones were prohibited entry. These same nurses were usually ones with great technical skill but weren't all that great with people. They preferred to give care without observers or anyone "in the way." And I also couldn't help but wonder if part of their attraction to the ICU was that most of their patients were on ventilators, unable to talk and were heavily sedated thus allowing them one hundred percent control.

The second group of nurses were polar opposites of the first group. They viewed the world in shades of grey and rarely saw things in black and white. Give them a paint-by-numbers project and they would probably toss it aside. Or if they did use it they would see the directions as mere suggestions. Coloring outside the lines describes their entire lifestyle yet they are able to reign themselves in enough to adhere to the most important rules. Patients and loved ones usually loved these nurses because they had good interpersonal skills, were friendly and outgoing and spent lots of time talking with them. They also interpreted visitation rules loosely, sometimes allowing non-family to visit and allowing visitors to remain around the clock. These easy going nurses often annoyed and frustrated their coworkers and managers who viewed their care as satisfactory but sloppy. Nurses who followed them (the next shift) resented the need to "clean up after them" and take care of overlooked details. They tended to clash with management more often than others, yet they knew their stuff, and usually provided good enough patient care to remain employed. They gave the appearance of being laid back and easy going, and didn't let much get to them. The exception was when one of the more controlling nurses tried to impose their rules and style. But for the most part, all the nurses left each other alone and each did their own thing except when teamwork was required for two or three person jobs and in emergencies.

The third group of nurses fell between the two extremes already described. They followed most, but not all rules. They had the common sense to identify the purpose and necessity (or not) of the rules in a given situation. They knew their stuff and provided very good care but knew when to not sweat the small stuff. If they had the chance to complete a paint-by-numbers project they might surprise you. One time they might follow the rules completely, yet ignore them another time. In most cases they would create a beautiful picture that adhered to the directions in some ways but were unique and creative in others. Nurses in this group recognized the intent of visitation rules and enforced them only when truly necessary. Examples usually included an emergency with the patient involved or the one next door. These nurses didn't allow just anyone at the patient's bedside, but understood that a marriage certificate wasn't the only consideration in determining who a significant other might be. Further they recognized that in most cases, it was beneficial for patient and family to allow at least one person to remain at the bed side most of the time. These nurses were actually the most flexible and were able to adapt to the styles and needs of others in order to get along and maintain high quality patient care.

I see myself in this last group. Depending upon the situation I can be a stickler for the rules, but most of the time I'm pretty flexible. I definitely go through life painting outside the lines much of the time, though not always. Unless their presence was disruptive in some way, I generally let family members take turns visiting the patient, spending as much time there as they wished. The only real exceptions were when that patient was undergoing procedures, or if there was an emergency next door. I didn't mind having family watch me or occasionally needing to work around them. It gave me valuable opportunities to explain to them the purpose of the equipment they saw and generally get to know them and the (often nonverbal) patient better. Family members usually voiced deep appreciation for this. Granted, I worked nights so the atmosphere was generally calmer with fewer people in the area than on day shift. Even so, when I later switched to day shift I still tried to follow the same philosophy. Many years later when my brother was the patient and I was the distraught family member, I knew I had done the right thing.

Many of my ICU patients were unconscious and on ventilators (breathing machines). While their condition might sometimes have impaired their hearing, I always operated on the assumption they could hear because it is known that hearing is the last sense people lose due to sedation, injury, or even when dying. Therefore, I was always careful to introduce myself, remind them where they were, and very simply, share what had led to their hospitalization. I reassured them I was going to take very good care of them, and always spoke gently before I touched them anywhere for any purpose. I simply assumed that if I were in their place that is how I would wish to be treated. From time to time, recovered patients later returned to thank us (which was very rewarding). They often made comments like, "I don't remember all your faces, but I do remember your voices."

One of the things I learned about myself during my time in the ICU is that I am not an adrenaline junkie. Each night I was happy to accept whatever patient(s) the charge nurse assigned me. If the patient was extremely critical and unstable, I rose to the challenge, but I didn't require this to feed a need for an adrenaline fix. I was just as content to care for the more stable patients so I could lavish as much TLC on them as I could. Oddly, my flexibility in this regard earned me the criticism of a few of my colleagues and the ICU Nursing Director on my annual review. She pointed out that "the other nurses have reported to me that you shy away from the more critical patients. You need to fight for the opportunity to take care of them just like the other nurses do."

I was dumbfounded. "Seriously?" I asked. "Are you kidding? You really want me to fight over patients with the other nurses?"

"Yes," she said, nodding her head. "That's how I know you are a real ICU nurse and deserve to work here."

I was literally speechless for a moment. I couldn't believe she thought this way and would actually say such a thing. Finally, I replied, "I totally disagree. The charge nurse is the leader and I believe the other nurses should accept whatever assignments they are given without argument unless there is an extremely good reason for it. I've been charge nurse on the medical unit and I know how demanding it can be. The last thing I needed was nurses who argued about assignments."

"Well this is the ICU," she said. "We do things differently here."

One of the most disturbing things about this event was that one of the nurses who accused me of shying away from complex patients had literally set me up, though I didn't see it at the time.

I was called to work one evening when the ICU had become very busy. Unlike the usual routine of giving report on the patient I was to take, the nurse had three charts laid out in front of me. "You get to choose!" she said, like I had won some sort of prize. "You can take these two, very nice, stable cardiac patients," she said as she pointed out two charts. "Or you can take this unstable, fresh, post-op patient." The patient had just undergone AAA repair. This is an aneurysm of the abdominal aorta which can be deadly if it ruptures. Repair is done to prevent this. But most patients were unhealthy beforehand and are often unstable afterwards. I had taken postop AAA patients before and was capable of taking the assignment. The interesting thing however, was the manner in which this nurse laid out my "choice." She made it extremely clear that she badly wanted to take the AAA patient. I considered her an excellent ICU nurse as well as one I would classify as an adrenaline junkie. She thrived on such challenges and it was clear that taking the AAA patient would be much more fun for her. I, on the other hand, was equally happy to take either assignment. Since she made it clear that letting her take the AAA patient would be doing her a great favor, I let her have him and I took the other assignment. She seemed thrilled as she went on her way. Yet when it came time for my annual review, she told a different version of the story to our Nursing Director making it sound like I was afraid of the AAA patient and had shied away from a challenging situation. This was hurtful to say the least and when I tried to explain the true nature of the interaction it was clear that my director believed her version.

Over the next several weeks it was obvious the charge nurses had been given specific instructions to assign me the most critical, least stable patients in the unit and observe my response. I could see them standing back to watch my reaction and judge my performance. I could only imagine what they had been told. I accepted the assignments as usual, without comment or complaint, and worked hard to provide the best care possible. I wasn't sure if their concern was genuine or if it was all another variation of how "nurses eat their young." This is an old, well-known, and (often) embarrassingly true saying that reveals how experienced nurses have become known for being especially hard on the newer nurses. Rather than mentoring and coaching them, as ought to be the case, they sometimes criticize and demoralize them, practically daring them to survive their early years in the profession. Only after they have satisfactorily proven themselves are the new nurses finally welcomed into the fold. What makes this even harder to believe is that the young nurses who suffered at the hand of the older ones often end up following their example.

I especially witnessed this later on in my role as a nurse educator when I took nursing students to the hospital. Getting the nurses there to work respectfully with students and to actually mentor them was one of the most challenging parts of my job. Thankfully not all nurses were or are this way. Some are natural educators and wonderful mentors. For them, my students and I were deeply grateful. We only wish the many others would follow their example.

After a time, it seems that I must have proven myself to the satisfaction of my director and things returned to normal. Interestingly, at my next annual review, she showered me with praise, saying, "I'm so pleased at your progress this past year. You've really proven yourself." Certainly, a year's worth of nursing provided opportunities for learning and growth so I wasn't going to argue the matter. Yet I knew that I had continued to conduct myself in the same manner as before and refused to ever fight over patients.

Expert Nurse

While working in ICU I also entered graduate school. The dual workload along with raising teenagers was extremely challenging. I did the very best I could. But like most women, I wanted to be all things to all people and in the process discovered that Super Woman is indeed a myth. I did my best given the time and resources available to me. But it was often stressful and I frequently felt stretched too thin. I learned and grew more than I can say, but very nearly burned myself out in the process.

Thankfully, I finished graduate school the spring of 1994 which was cause for celebration and a huge relief to my family and me. Oddly the same nursing director and co-workers who accused me of avoiding challenges in the ICU also failed to provide support, encouragement, or even comment on my educational achievement. I earned a master's degree in nursing (MSN) as a Family Nurse Practitioner. Most people would consider this quite a challenge and an excellent way to stretch oneself.

I knew from the outset, that I would not likely work as a FNP. I was much more interested in writing, research, and education and figured the FNP degree provided a great foundation to work from. Though I was unsure how it would all play out I was confident that it would. This proved to be true.

The remainder of my nursing practice included a year at a private vocational-rehabilitation firm as a nurse consultant, a year back at the hospital in the float pool, followed by another eleven years in the Medical/Oncology float pool. Returning to my original nursing home on that unit, I became aware of how much I had learned and grown during my time away. My physical examination skills had improved significantly and I was noting things I suspected I might have missed in the past. For example, I frequently heard heart murmurs and other abnormal heart sounds that (according to documentation) were missed by many other nurses, and even some physicians. I could also envision my patients' cardiac rhythms as I listened to their hearts and often knew what they would look like on a heart monitor. My understanding of the causes behind my patients' disease processes was much more solid and my understanding of how the medications worked was more accurate. I had also grown in my ability to communicate effectively with patients and their loved ones. There were a thousand other things I noticed that reassured me that I was indeed on the road to developing the nursing expertise I'd always wanted. As I considered the next direction for my career, I remembered how much I had enjoyed working with students and knew I now had more to offer them. Therefore, it felt like time to leave full-time staff nursing and enter the world of education.

Becoming a Nurse Educator

Unbeknownst to me, my teaching career actually began as soon as I began working as a staff nurse. Nurses teach patients every day but don't often think of it as teaching. Yet it is, and it's quite important. We teach patients how to use their medications, how to perform wound care, how to use medical devices, how to modify their diet, and a thousand other things.

As a staff nurse I'd had the opportunity to work with nursing students from the local community college when they came to the hospital for their clinical rotations. Sadly, not all nurses enjoy this. But I loved it. It felt great to share what I knew with them and to show them the various techniques I'd developed for completing so many of my nursing duties in a timely manner. I also discovered a passion for teaching students how to provide patient care in a manner I believed upheld high quality standards and also treated patients with dignity and compassion. I liked being able to influence future nurses in a manner I believed would have a positive impact on their future and the well-being of their future patients. I wanted to do more with students but was limited by the constraints of my role as a hospital employee and my lack of a master's degree. At the time, I recall the college instructor saying that I should consider graduate school so I could teach full time. I shrugged it off then, yet eventually decided that perhaps she was right. In the meantime I decided to inquire at the college to see if I might be able to be a clinical instructor on a part-time basis. I figured it would be a good way to try on the educator hat before making a larger commitment.

I taught clinical on a part-time basis over the next several years along with my work as a staff nurse. I sacrificed income and benefits to do this. Yet the combination was ideal from a professional standpoint. Working as an educator strengthened my knowledge base and skill performance which made me a better staff nurse. Working as a staff nurse provided more "real world" experience which made me a better educator. The responsibility of teaching students provided a huge incentive for making sure that I knew and taught the correct way to do things.

Over time, I taught first and second year students in several clinical locations. My favorite was taking students to the Medical/Oncology unit of my hospital where I knew the ropes and the staff. But I also had the opportunity to stretch myself and my comfort zone by taking students to local nursing homes and a small rural hospital. In every case I'm sure I learned as much as my students. I also gained a deep respect for what nurses do in these settings. Like other hospital nurses I had developed a rather smug attitude and believed we were the "best" and in some ways the only "real" nurses. I thought nurses in long term care (nursing homes), clinics, or small rural hospitals were less challenged and therefore less knowledgeable and less skilled. Boy was I wrong. Because the setting is different, the skill set is sometimes different. Yet I was to learn that the challenges, though different, were equal to, or sometimes even greater than what I was used to.

Program Director

Eventually, after completing my master's degree, I decided I would very much like to be a full-time college educator. However, there were no full-time positions available and it appeared as if there wouldn't be for quite some time. Yet, at that time, our college had decided to offer a new Medical Assistant program. Therefore, they were looking for someone to develop the program, run it, and be the primary educator. I considered the position initially but did not apply because my goal was to be a nurse educator.

In the meantime, the interview committee interviewed numerous candidates without offering the job to any. As the position remained unfilled, and time passed, I was asked by a college administrator to consider applying. This caused me to carefully reconsider my earlier decision. Ultimately I applied, was interviewed, and was hired for the job. It turned out to be a rich learning experience. However, I was quite naïve about what I was getting into. They literally handed me a medical assisting textbook with a brief list of courses to be taught and said, "Congratulations! Your first class begins in two weeks."

If I had it to do over I would still have accepted the position, but I would have negotiated for more prep time. As I eventually learned, two weeks is barely enough time to prepare even one course. I had four the first quarter, and an average of four more for each of the three following quarters. I had to quickly educate myself before I could begin educating my students. I worked seven days a week, nearly every waking hour for the next two years. Regardless of what the college calendar said, there were no vacations for me. The saving grace was that I absolutely loved it. I was crazy busy, yet I recall thinking "I can't believe they are paying me to do this! I'd almost do it for free!" That's how I knew I'd landed just where I was supposed to be.

By the end of the third year, not only could I describe what a certified medical assistant (CMA) is, but I could also articulate why, in certain situations, they might be a more versatile and valued employee than a nurse. Furthermore, I had developed the full curriculum, taught most of the courses, developed working relationships with most of the healthcare employers in the area (for clinical rotations), conducted and wrote the program Self Study Report, and led the entire process through which the program earned national accreditation. Yet what I was most proud of was the four graduated classes who earned their CMA credentials and became successful employees of many of the area's healthcare employers. My favorite part was watching their personal growth and transformation. They entered as insecure students and grew into competent, confident professionals with a solid knowledge base and a valuable skill set which made them highly desirable employees and capable wage earners. Completing the program literally changed most of their lives and I was proud to be a part of that process.

After several years as the Medical Assistant Program Director, a full-time nursing faculty position became available. Initially I felt conflicted about whether to apply. It was what I had long wanted. Yet I had invested so much of myself into the MA program and did not want to desert it. I knew I could only leave it if I felt it was in good hands. Fortunately, there were several great candidates and the one that was hired has done an excellent job.

Full-Time Nurse Educator

Switching gears to become a full-time nursing educator was easy in some respects since first and foremost I had always been a nurse and I had taught clinical nursing for years. Yet in other ways it required an even deeper commitment to continuing education because, once again, I felt a huge responsibility to teach things correctly. Our ultimate responsibility was to produce graduates ready to work as nurses with entry-level nursing skills and knowledge. Yet what employers always seemed to want were highly skilled, confident nurses with the proficiency that only comes with several years of work experience. They often seemed to have forgotten they too had been novices once. This left a huge gap between our reality and their expectations. And the gap threatened to widen on a daily basis as the profession of nursing continually grew in scope. To bridge this gap and remain relevant we continually sought ways to improve the program, teach more effectively, and better prepare students for the workplace. The pressure was always on educators and students as we were constantly expected to function at higher and higher levels. This resulted in an intense, challenging program known for being difficult and demanding.

While all of this was happening we were also under pressure from college administrators. They wanted us to somehow guarantee that all students would pass all courses, pass the NCLEX exam after graduation, and go on to become excellent nurses. We wanted this as badly as they did, probably more so. However, we recognized the critical imperative of maintaining adequate standards to ensure current and future patient safety. Not being nurses themselves, the administrators sometimes failed to understand why we occasionally appeared to be stubborn and unyielding in this regard. They only saw the students at hand. We saw the students and their patients. We knew the potential repercussions if a student made an error in the dosage or administration of a medication or any one of a thousand other potential mistakes. We didn't want that on anyone's conscience; the students', ours, or the college's as a whole. And we certainly didn't want the patient or their loved ones to suffer from an avoidable mistake. Because of this we were fairly strict in our standards for both classroom and clinical performance.

I learned so many valuable lessons during my years as an educator; more than I can write about. However, one of the earliest came in the wise words of a more experienced colleague who stated one day, "We don't give students their grades. They earn them." And I realized how true it was. My coworkers and I did everything possible to support student success, but ultimately it was up to students to come to class, study the material, do the work, and earn their passing scores. Similarly, they were responsible for showing up at clinical on time, fully prepared to provide safe patient care that met the nursing standards. If they did so, they succeeded. And if not, well, they didn't.

Another important lesson was that it was much more important for students to learn from me than it was for them to like me. This was a difficult lesson at first. Like most people I wanted to be liked. I liked being liked. It feels good and makes life pleasant. However, I ultimately had to realize that I hadn't been hired to be liked. I had been hired to teach. I ultimately realized that student learning was the number one goal. Coming to this realization allowed me to maintain program standards, and when necessary, to confront students regarding unsafe or unprofessional behavior. And ultimately I realized the most meaningful compliment students could give was not about how much they liked me. Rather it was about how much they learned from me.

This was and is an area that many educators struggle with. They mistake being liked for being a good teacher. Consequently, they are sometimes afraid to confront students about their inappropriate behavior. I saw this in a few of my colleagues. Sadly, it sometimes resulted in their choosing to overlook unacceptable student behaviors and left it up to the rest of us to be the "mean" ones who would confront it. This was one of my greatest frustrations when it came to teamwork. I felt that students deserved consistency from all educators, whether full-time or part-time. Teammates who failed to do their part not only let me down, but ultimately let students down as well.

Having said that, I must also say that working as a team with many of my fellow instructors was also one of my greatest joys. We each had different areas of expertise and very different personality types. This made for an intensely rich learning environment in which we were all learners and we were all teachers amongst our faculty group. As we worked together I developed great respect for each of them. As an added bonus I developed close friendships with some of them as well.

Learning Styles

I'm sure there were hundreds of lessons along my path as a nurse educator, but the last one I will mention is what I discovered about student learning styles. A student's learning style, described simply, is the manner in which a given student most effectively learns. One of my deepest regrets as an educator is that I didn't come to appreciate the value of understanding learning styles until the last couple of years that I taught.

Many informational articles regarding learning styles are available online, some easier to understand than others. There are a number of different approaches and philosophies regarding learning styles which can be confusing for students and teachers alike. For my own use I decided that the simpler and easier philosophies were also the most "user friendly." For this reason, I decided to use the one that was built around our senses: sight, touch, hearing and so on. Examples of these styles include visual (sight), auditory (sound), and kinesthetic (touch) learners. In addition to use of the senses, most learners also fall into the categories of being either solitary (individual) or social (interactive) learners. As I came to understand the key styles, I located a simple online test for my students to use so they could identify their own unique style. Everyone is a blend of all styles, yet most of us gravitate more to one or two particular areas. Once students began to better understand how they most effectively learned, they could modify their study strategies so as to waste less time on ineffective techniques and more time on the ones that were most effective for them. To illustrate the usefulness of understanding one's learning style I will tell you a story about one of my students.

Alex

Alex was a kind, friendly student who struggled terribly the first time she took the pharmacology course and sadly, did not pass. A year or two later she returned to retake the class in hopes of passing so she could continue the nursing program. When I heard she was returning I was concerned because I wanted her to experience success. If feeling like a failure once is hard, twice can be totally devastating.

I had recently been learning more about student learning styles and was pondering how to incorporate the information into my teaching. As I'd feared, Alex scored poorly on the first exam. But fortunately she came to see me afterward. I shared with her some of what I'd learned about learning styles and then we identified her style. Next we identified possible learning strategies she could use to improve her chances of success. I was happy to see that she scored significantly higher on the next exam and I wondered what study strategies she had used. A few days later she came by my office and told me the story.

Alex had two assignments looming over her head. One was to prepare for a pharmacology exam and the other was a painting for her art class. As she considered the two assignments and our conversation about learning styles she developed the following strategy. She chose to study alone knowing that she was a solitary learner. She also knew she was most strongly visual, with kinesthetic and auditory tied for second place. This meant that any activities involving strong images, pictures, diagrams, and such along with use of sound and physical movement should be helpful. So she set up her canvas and paints, laid out her pharmacology text book on a table close by, and had recorded lectures from class on hand as well as some of her favorite music. She alternated playing the taped lecture and looking at her class notes and visuals from the text book, all while she painted. When she tired of listening to lectures she played music as she committed certain data to memory, all while still painting and even "writing" data in the air with her paintbrush. The result was that she successfully completed her art assignment and felt better prepared for the pharmacology exam than any time previously. As she took the exam, she said she could see in her mind's eye the information she painted on the canvas or drew in the air. She could even hear some of the lecture pieces or music that had become associated with certain data in her mind. This helped a great deal with recall. She was beyond excited at how well it had worked and for the first time she felt hopeful that she could succeed at her chosen career. I was nearly as excited as she and for the first time I fully realized the powerful role learning styles could play in student success. After that experience I devoted more time and energy to helping my students identify their learning styles and brainstorming study strategies.

About the same time as this, I was working on the second edition of my first book "Medical Terminology in a Flash!"[3] In response to requests from many of our educator-adopters, I was adding more of this very content to the book so they and their students all over the country could use it as well. As a now retired educator, my hope is that they take and use this information to the fullest possible extent. At one time I paid lip service to the new buzzwords about learning styles. Now I am a true believer and hope that other educators will continue to help students learn and study in ways that are best for them as individuals.

From Nurse to Patient

Making the transition from nurse and nurse educator to patient has been one of the greatest challenges I've ever faced. In the beginning it was a decidedly uncomfortable place to be. But some of the very students I supported in learning and transforming into nurses have in return provided me with some of the most meaningful support I've experienced. They gave of their valuable time and energy in ways I never expected to let me know they cared. To know they are now working in my community caring for those who live here, leaves me feeling comforted and proud. And as I've had time to process and accept my new role as patient, I've decided it almost feels right. It's like I've come full circle and have been able to take full advantage of the rich learning to be had on both sides of this fence.

Chapter 3 Notes

1. Donna Wilk Cardillo, copyright 2017 nursetheory.com http://www.nursetheory.com/nursing-quotes/

2. Northwest Medstar Critical Care Transport Service, October 28, 2015, https://www.nwmedstar.org/ (accessed 3/25/2017). MedStar was formed in 1994 with the merging of Spokane's Heartflight and Lifebird programs.

3. Sharon Eagle, *Medical Terminology in a Flash! A Multiple Learning Styles Approach* (Philadelphia: F.A. Davis, 2011) 2nd edition, 2015.

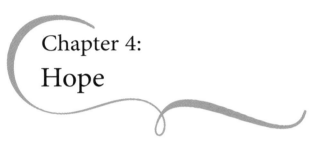

Chapter 4:
Hope

Hope. It's the only thing stronger than fear.[1]

The Right to Hope

I am hopeful that the remainder of my life will be meaningful as I seek to achieve the purposes God has for me. I also hope for a peaceful, pain-free transition when it's my time to die. And I have great hope for a meaningful existence afterwards. To accept the inevitability of my own death does not mean I have given up all hope. It means I am embracing a different dimension of hope. I do not believe death is the end. In fact, I believe there is much more to come.

I would also support anyone who feels that it's not their time to die. I agree with Dr. Jerome Groopman who states that patients have the right to determine when they will relinquish hope for a physical cure. To retain hope and maintain autonomy prevents patients from feeling helpless.[2] In the medical and legal worlds autonomy refers to the patient's right to free, informed choice. To make such choices they must fully understand their options and the probable consequences of each. Furthermore, they must believe their wishes have been heard, accepted, respected, and acted upon.

If they still hold out hope for a cure or at least a remission that buys more time here on planet Earth, they are entitled to all the support and help they can possibly muster.

I only hope they are doing it for themselves and not out of a sense of obligation or guilt. This statement is based upon years of experience where I've seen family and loved ones pushing the patient saying, "fight," "hold on," or "don't give up" when the patient is clearly exhausted and ready to go. Often when I spoke with the patient in private, they confided in me that they felt exhausted and ready to die but feared letting down their family, friends, or even their doctors. Ellen was one such patient.

Ellen

I was working night shift in the ICU in the early nineties. One night I had a seventy-four-year-old woman who had been admitted with complications of diabetes. Over the previous twenty years, she had undergone so many amputations that she was now left with nothing remaining of either leg. She had non-healing wounds from her last surgery in spite of aggressive wound care and antibiotic therapy. She was scheduled for surgery the next morning. It would be an uncommon and aggressive form of amputation that would remove parts of her buttocks and lower torso.

It was a relatively calm night in the ICU which gave me the luxury of spending time with Ellen and Barb, her forty-eight-year-old daughter, who sat at her bedside. As they talked I noted some hesitation on Ellen's part when she spoke about the scheduled surgery. Her daughter also questioned the surgical plan but wanted to support her mother. As I listened to Ellen I heard her repeat, more than once, that she didn't want to let her doctor down because "he had been trying so very hard" to help her. I had worked with this physician enough to know that he was the sort that took death as a personal failure so it made sense to me that he would be encouraging her to not give up.

As we talked through the night I was careful to make only positive comments about her physician. However, I also pointed out, "He's a big boy and can take care of himself. It's your job to take care of yourself. You have every right to voice your own wants and needs. If that means undergoing surgery, then you are in good hands. But you need to make this decision for yourself, not for anyone else." As she and her daughter talked about it throughout the night, Ellen reached the conclusion that she did not wish to have the surgery after all. Her daughter fully supported her and I could sense the relief they both felt. I told them they must be sure to tell her physician this as soon as they saw him. I also relayed the information in shift report to the oncoming nurse so that she could continue to support them.

Returning to work a few days later I encountered Barb in the hospital entrance. Upon seeing me, she immediately embraced me and tearfully thanked me for what I "did" for her mother. She said they both felt at peace about the decision they had made. After talking with the physician, her mom was transferred out of ICU and into a hospice room on another floor. She described their last few days together as "precious" and stated her mother had "died peacefully" that very afternoon. She further expressed how thankful she was that her mother had avoided yet another surgery and all that went with it. She added, "Mom was at peace and ready to go." As I reflected on the experience over the next few days I wondered how anyone could call Ellen's death a "failure."

∾

I've had many conversations with patients in which I encouraged them to give themselves permission to be more honest with family and physician about what they really wanted. I've had equally as many conversations with family and loved ones, encouraging them to abandon small talk for real talk about what matters most. To speak of love and appreciation and, when appropriate, share the final greatest gift they could bestow, which is to give their loved one "permission to go" if that is what is needed. Very often grateful family members thanked me afterwards. They knew the conversation was necessary but didn't know how to get there. As it turns out all they needed was a gentle push and "permission" from the nurse.

The Hope Club?

Hearing that I had terminally advanced cancer felt unreal and it took quite a long time to sink in. I've always been a realist and never expected to live forever. Even so, having cancer was a difficult concept to wrap my brain around. The voices in my head continued to argue with one another for quite some time about what was real and what I wished was real.

Once my diagnosis was confirmed I found myself sitting in the Radiation-Oncology waiting room five days a week for two weeks. The room was filled with other cancer patients, some bald, some wearing scarves or wigs, some still looking fairly healthy, and others obviously in the later stages of their disease. The latter, given away by their dark, sunken eyes, emaciated bodies, and slightly yellow- or green-tinged skin. I recall once seeing a young woman who might have been in her early twenties. She was completely bald, very thin, and frail in appearance. Her pale skin had the light greenish cast I had seen in cancer patients before. She leaned for support against a man who I assumed was her father. That she felt weak and ill was obvious and I recall thinking that she didn't have long to live. I knew the look and I felt bad for all she had been through and was still going through. I found myself even wondering why she was there. Death couldn't be far off, yet here she was waiting her turn for another radiation treatment. Did she still feel a sense of hope? Was she holding on, hoping for a cure? Was she trying to buy a bit more time? Was she doing it for herself or for family? Perhaps this was merely a palliative treatment, designed to relieve related symptoms rather than cure.

As hard as it sometimes was to look at these members of my new club, I also found myself feeling a certain kinship, a sort of comfort, being in their presence, because I knew that they knew how I felt. I was sad for them, yet glad to feel that I was not totally alone. I wanted to reach out and talk to some of them, to somehow bridge the divide created by the etiquette of silence demanded by most medical waiting rooms. But I didn't know how and didn't want to intrude or cause offense. So I sat in silence each day, waiting my turn. I never saw the young woman again.

I've seen other patients since that day. Many others. Some young, but most probably around my age or older. I've wondered about their stories. Were they as shocked as I when their physician told them they had cancer? The fact that they were undergoing treatment led me to assume they were feeling some degree of hope. If I asked them to define it, I wondered what they would say. And what specifically were they hoping for? A cure? More time? To live until Christmas (my hope that first year)? Or were they daring enough to hope for many Christmases? Was there a daughter to walk down the aisle? A new grandchild to be held? A golden anniversary to celebrate? What enabled them to continue on with hope, week after week? I also wondered how their spiritual beliefs, if any, impacted how they felt. Had they considered what dying and death might be like? I know I had. I couldn't imagine not thinking about it. What did they hope would happen? Does hope only allow expectation of a cure? If one has accepted the impending reality of death then is he or she, by definition, now without hope? Or are we allowed to hope for things other than a cure without being accused of having given up?

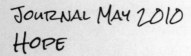

JOURNAL MAY 2010
HOPE

Can one hope for hope? This may sound silly and redun-
dant but I'm serious. I do have hope. But I wouldn't mind
having even more. There is something empowering about it.
Without it, like plants without water, we tend to wither and
die. It's the driving force that helps us get out of bed each day,
helps us to dream, and to identify and achieve our goals. It
keeps us moving forward in the face of adversity, helps us get
back on our feet in the face of failure and enables us to cheer
on those around us.

Defining Hope

Most of us have some idea what hope does for us. But few of us
can clearly define it. This got me to wondering; what is it really? I
checked a number of resources and found there was no one distinct
definition yet all were similar. Most sources define hope as a feeling or belief that what is desired is likely to occur. There seems to
be an element of faith involved; faith that things will work out for
the best.

Fundamentally, hope is empowering and seems vital to life.
Without it, we wither like plants without water. Yet I would argue
that hope can also provide peace and serenity as we move toward
death. Hope can help us accept this inevitable transition in which
we are relieved from bodily suffering and our spiritual selves are
free to move forward into our next adventure.

Dr. Groopman describes hope as the "elevating feeling" we have
when we anticipate a "better future."[3] He further states that hope
provides both the bravery and ability to confront and overcome life's

challenges and believes it's as important to his patients as any procedure or medication he might prescribe. Years of practice led him to
appreciate the significance of hope in the lives of his patients, making
all the difference in their ability to recover (or not). On a personal
level he found that hope impacted his own physical and emotional
health and gave him the power he needed to overcome nearly twenty
years of chronic pain. During his lifelong practice treating patients
with various forms of cancer, he came to understand that hope was
available to them only when they had free choice. Cathleen Fanslow-
Brunjes said that hope is one of the three basic needs of the dying
along with the need for self-expression and the need to know they
will not be abandoned.[4] She further states that hope motivates change
whether the individual transitions into death, or another manner of
living. I appreciate this because it acknowledges that hope can ease a
person across the threshold of death into whatever comes next, which
is one of the key points of this book.

Hopeful people might be described as assured, serene, buoyant,
confident, and full of faith,[5] whereas hopeless people might be seen
as despairing, discouraged, useless, or depressed.[6] Both examples
sound extreme but anyone might be anywhere on a continuum
between the two.

Journal October 2010
More Thoughts on Hope

I wonder if hope is what's missing for people who suffer
severe, chronic depression. Maybe that's why depression
hasn't been a problem for me (thus far). Sometimes I feel very
sad, but that isn't the same thing as feeling depressed. Even
when I feel very sad I still feel a great sense of hope.

For many of us, hope is fueled by our faith. And perhaps our faith is fueled by hope. I think they are intertwined in ways I don't fully understand. When I recall the many patients I cared for at the end of life, I noticed dramatic differences between those with hope and faith and those without. Those without often presented with signs of depression, such as being withdrawn and tearful. But there was more to it. For many there was fear; fear of the dying process and fear of the unknown. This sometimes resulted in a desperation to hold on to life as if the inevitable could somehow be prevented. Some were overcome with regrets about mistakes made, relationships not reconciled, wounds left open. For some there was a deep, dark anger. It was sometimes a mask for their fear. But sometimes it seemed a genuine anger directed toward God, family, and even the nurses providing their care.

In most cases I was able to maintain my caring, professional presence. I knew it wasn't personal. Yet at times, I'm sorry to say, I found myself feeling hurt and frustrated. Here I was, the one who was with them at the end, doing everything in my power to help them feel cared for and comfortable, yet because I was the one who was there, I was an easy target, and at times received the brunt of their anger. I noticed I was more inclined to feel this way when I was exhausted and my own reserves were low.

I did everything in my power to provide comfort and encourage hope and faith. I offered chaplain services or sometimes brought in their own pastor or priest. I listened (as much as time allowed) when they felt like talking. I shared my own faith if they asked, but was careful not to push. I took measures to relieve pain and anxiety and provide comfort. But for these patients it seemed I could never do enough. I suspected they were dying in the same manner as they had lived. Such folks usually held tightly to their anger, fear, and hatred for though it provided no comfort, it was all they had.

Martha was such a patient. She had been something of a frequent flyer during most of the time I worked there. She was exceptionally needy; she pushed her call bell incessantly and expected the nurse to be in her room at all times. She knew we had other patients to care for but seemed unable to feel empathy or concern for them or for anyone but herself. She accepted physical care but resisted any form of emotional or spiritual care. Neither was she interested in any sort of problem solving. It was as if she wanted to be miserable because it was her comfort zone. When the nurses tried to provide a therapeutic presence and listen to her concerns all she did was complain about how miserable her life had been and how uncaring and ungrateful her family members were. She was extremely repetitive and her favorite saying was "After everything I did for them, you'd think they would be more grateful!"

After a time, it became difficult to listen to. She predicted her own demise on every stay, for years on end. In all the time she was there I never saw family or visitors of any kind. This begged the question: were they really as uncaring and awful as she made them out to be, or had she driven them away with her negative behavior? Eventually her prediction came true and she died alone, except for the nurse at her side.

I am glad to say there were many patients full of faith and hope. Once again I did everything in my power to provide care and comfort. Yet with such people I often felt that they gave more to me than I gave to them. They were an inspiration to everyone who came into contact with them. Their hearts were full of love and gratitude for the lives they had lived and for those around them. They were notable for their absence of fear and I could often feel a tangible sense of peace when I entered their rooms. Occasionally they felt anxiety but their coping skills were strong and it was usually short-lived. Their family and loved ones were often the same way and they provided an awesome support system for one another.

June was such a patient. When I admitted her to my unit one

day I was surprised to see that she was there for end-of-life care. The reason for my surprise was that she was so cheerful and upbeat that upon first impression, I mistook how ill she was. As it turned out she had a type of leukemia that was deadly. The doctor estimated she would live for two weeks at the time of her diagnosis one week earlier. She had chosen to enter the hospital for hospice care to relieve her family from the burden of her care. June was friendly, warm, gracious, and thankful for every little thing I did for her. Once she was settled in bed I recall her looking at me and asking, "So how long is this going to take?"

I wasn't quite sure what she meant and sought clarification "How long is what going to take?" I asked.

"Dying," she said. "I'm ready to get on with it, and I'm hoping it won't take long." There was no fear or anxiety on her face. Instead she had an expression of expectation and excitement. She was ready to go and was looking forward to her journey. That she was much beloved became evident later that day as family, friends, and well-wishers began stopping by. There were tears, but the atmosphere was not sad. It was more like a going away party and everyone who loved her wanted to pay one more visit before she left. She was overflowing with hope and her faith was nearly tangible. She fully believed she was embarking on the ultimate journey and knew she was saying, "See you later," rather than, "Goodbye," to her loved ones.

Although I do not fully understand the hope/faith connection, I do agree with author Henri Nouwen, who shares that hope and faith are more about the One we have faith and hope in than about using a shallow form of faith as a means to get the things we want in life.[7] He points out that true hope (and faith) aren't focused on things or even outcomes but are an attitude of openness toward God trusting that He is working for my greater good.[8] Hope and trust are in Him and my prayers are directed, not toward the gifts I wish to receive but toward Him.

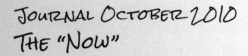

Journal October 2010
The "Now"

Am I making the most of the time I have left? How does one really do that? I try to spend time with loved ones and cherish each moment. I find myself wanting to stop the clock, to just hold certain moments in time and make them last. Yet no matter what I do, the clock keeps ticking, moments pass, and the "now" becomes a memory. I want to hold onto it but don't know how. So instead I create and collect precious memories with my loved ones knowing that one day I will be gone and they will be left with the memories. I know from experience that memories just aren't enough when you are longing for someone. But sometimes they are all we have and are the best we can do. Perhaps the clock will stop in the next life and the passage of time will be meaningless. But for now, time marches on. So I pray that the memories we create and collect will be precious and meaningful and will provide some comfort to those I love.

Chapter 4 Notes

1. Suzanne Collins, *The Hunger Games.* Scholastic Press, New York, 2008. Kindle locations 1121-1122.

2. Groopman, Jerome, *Anatomy of Hope: How People Prevail in the Face of Illness.* Random House, New York, 2004. Kindle location 336-345.

3. Ibid. Kindle location 42.

4. Cathleen Fanslow-Brunjes, *Using the Power of Hope to Cope with Dying: The Four Stages of Hope.* Quill Driver Books, Fresno, 2008. Kindle location 573.

5. Thesaurus.com. Roget's 21st Century Thesaurus, Third Edition. Philip Lief Group 2009. http://www.thesaurus.com/browse/hopeful (accessed 3/29/2017).

6. Thesaurus.com. Roget's 21st Century Thesaurus, Third Edition. Philip Lief Group 2009. http://www.thesaurus.com/browse/hopeless (accessed 3/29/2017).

7. Henri Nouwen. *With Open Hands.* Ava Marie Press, Indiana, 2006. p. 73-74.

Chapter 5:
The God Connection

But those who hope in the Lord will renew their strength.
They will soar on wings like eagles;
They will run and not grow weary, They will walk and not faint.[1]

There is a difference between sharing my religious chronology and my spiritual beliefs. But to understand the latter, you must know something of the former.

My spiritual beliefs have evolved as a part of my life-long journey, rather than as a result of any one event in time. During my early years my mother took my siblings and me to the United Methodist Church where we learned the basics about Christianity by attending Sunday school. We also attended summer Vacation Bible School at a different denomination church within walking distance from our house. I didn't realize it at the time, but my mother's willingness to do this let us know that we could learn about God and Jesus equally well in any Christian church denomination. One wasn't necessarily any better or more "right" than another. This was a valuable lesson and has had a lasting influence on me. My family moved several times over the next few years and we ended up living in town where I was able to walk to most activities. I began visiting several different types of churches to see which one was the best fit for me. An Assembly of God church, just two blocks away from my house was in the middle of a big summer revival. I decided to try it out and before I knew it I had been "saved" and was faithfully attending their nightly meetings. It was quite exciting but in all honesty I wasn't entirely sure what it really meant. I thought I had been a Christian before that so I wasn't entirely sure what I had been saved from, although my AG friends told me my prior experiences hadn't really counted. I wasn't sure how I felt about that. After a short time, the novelty wore off and I realized the AG church wasn't a good fit for me. However, I did believe that I had taken a step closer to God through my experiences there and it left me wanting more.

Throughout high school I attended two churches. The United Methodist was my comfort zone and I enjoyed my involvement in the youth group there. I made several very good friends who are still in my life today. Yet I sometimes felt that I needed something more. A very close friend attended the Nazarene church. Throughout high school we practically lived at each other's houses so it felt natural to begin attending church with her as well. This involvement influenced my college choice and after graduation we left home together to attend a Nazarene college in Idaho.

I learned more about God and Christianity through both churches over these years. As a result, my own personal relationship with God slowly grew as well. But I always found myself questioning what was truly of God and what was just a part of church doctrine. I couldn't help but notice the basic tenets of faith were the same at each. Yet there were differences in the details and some big differences in the "rules." From what I could tell, these "rules" came from church doctrine, created by church leaders, and not from the bible. This created feelings of ambivalence on my part and I soon developed a resistance for anything that seemed to be a man-made rule and not a genuine part of the faith. For example, I loved the Nazarene church and my friends there. I also loved the college I attended for nearly two years. Yet I found myself frustrated with so many of their rules for behavior. For example, two key rules that impacted my age group prohibited us from dancing or attending movies. And though it was explained to me numerous times, I failed to understand how such rules could be commands from God. I loved music and loved to dance. I also grew up going to movies and couldn't imagine ever giving that up. Being a teenager who loved to socialize, these rules felt too restrictive for me. After nearly two years there, I began to feel stifled and realized that the Nazarene church wasn't a good fit for me either. I began praying for and looking for something else.

About this time, a Christmas vacation out of state to visit another close friend influenced the direction of my life and introduced me to yet another church. It was a non-denominational church with a very large number of people my age, a strong music program and a large, very active choir. These features deeply attracted me and I felt this was where I was destined to be. I withdrew from college and moved there a few weeks later at the end of the term.

I attended this church for eight years, met and married my first husband and had my three children during that time. When I reflect back on that time it is with feelings of great ambivalence. I made some good friends there and became involved in the choir for a time. This provided opportunities to learn a great deal about self-discipline and team work. We traveled around the Pacific Northwest and in 1976 to Europe and Israel. This was all (mostly) great fun. The overseas trip was one I'd never have otherwise been able to make and became one of the highlights of my life. In this church I also developed an appreciation and love for Israel and the Jewish people in general. I think this has been a good thing in my life but please don't mistake it to mean that I have any less respect for other peoples or religions. There was plenty of biblical teaching that seemed great at the time. But since then I've found myself needing to sort what was valid and useful from what was not. Just one example would be the teaching that women should be submissive to our husbands in all things and to men in general. Perhaps this worked for some of the members. But for me it served to emphasize and worsen some very real problems in my marriage.

After I'd spent approximately six years in the church it erupted in scandal. The financial manager was accused of embezzlement and, after a lengthy and much publicized trial, was found "not guilty." However most church members I talked with believed differently. So did I. There were other accusations against him as well as against the head pastor. To this day I have no idea which ones might have been true. What did become clear to me as all the dirty laundry was aired was many of the unethical practices. Everyone was pressured to give money. I later learned that certain individuals had actually been instructed to take out personal loans and give the money to the church. The leadership was accused of playing matchmaker among many of the young adults. Yet in some cases they interfered with relationships and prohibited marriage. There were many weddings. Short engagements were encouraged so as to reduce temptation for premarital sex. There was more but I have no desire to share it all. I only share these things to explain why I became so angry and disillusioned and finally left the church.

I continued to feel angry for many years and stayed away from church because of it. I was not angry with God. I was angry with those who professed to serve Him by manipulating others to meet their own needs. I also wondered how I could have been so naïve as to have missed it all. With hindsight I began to realize that there had been clues about much of it but between being a good (submissive) church member and the sort who always wanted to believe the best about people, I had managed to somehow overlook it all. When the truth came out, I felt betrayed and resentful. But I also learned some valuable lessons. One was that no church should ever function that independently. Churches that are part of denominations (Baptist, Methodist, Catholic, etc.), must be responsible to them and follow guidelines for money and resource management. There are also codes of conduct for leadership which helps keep individuals from misusing church funds or manipulating church members for personal gain.

The other big lesson for me was that I am responsible for my own beliefs and behavior. I vowed that I would never again let another person, regardless of title or position, do my spiritual thinking or decision making for me or claim to know "God's will" for me again.

During the next year my marriage ended and I avoided church for many years thereafter. I was averse to anything that reminded me of the bad experiences I'd had and I was therefore reluctant to put my faith and trust in any form of church leadership. But contrary to what many of my friends thought, I never stopped believing in God. My problem wasn't with Him. It was with those who claimed to serve Him by deceiving and using others for personal gain.

I continued to seek God on my own through an active prayer life, lots of reading and conversations with others. I still considered myself a believer but wasn't sure if I still fit the description of being a "Christian." I went through a time of deep reflection and truth-seeking. I questioned virtually everything I had ever been taught and underwent a sort of "sorting process" where I pondered and evaluated what felt authentic and valuable versus what didn't. As I did this, I held onto the former and discarded the latter. What I was left with began to form the foundation of my new belief system.

Eventually I felt the desire to return to church but struggled to identify a church home where I felt free to be myself and question the status quo. It took a long time but eventually I made peace with the notion that there is no perfect church. This enabled me to identify a place where I feel supported in my growing process which includes sometimes questioning and even disagreeing with stated church doctrine. Health issues have prevented regular attendance but I feel included and supported by the pastor, which I appreciate.

So what, exactly, do I now believe? My beliefs have been evolving my entire life so I can only describe what I believe now knowing that it may be slightly different next week or next year. Yet the place I've landed really isn't so very far from where I first started. First and foremost, I believe in God, the creator, greater power and a father figure although my understanding is that God includes both masculine and feminine energy. I also believe in Jesus but have questioned for many years what his relationship is to other religious leaders like Buddha, Mohammed, and others. After careful thought and deliberation, I rejected, several years ago, the notion that only Christians go to heaven and everyone else goes to hell. I've come to understand God as a loving father who desires that all of His children would eventually be with Him. Therefore, it simply makes no sense to me that He would have created a circumstance in which ninety percent don't make it. I wouldn't have. I love my three children more than life itself. I would never create ground rules that would exclude two of them.

I believe that knowing God is the goal and various religions are vehicles that people use to reach Him. While we may call Him by different names I think we are all seeking the same one true God. For this reason, I believe I will see people from other faiths when I go to heaven. My entire life I've felt something within me that has always sought to identify and know God. I was born into a Christian family, so I've used Christianity as my vehicle to reach out to Him. But I could as easily have been born in another country where I was raised in a Buddhist, Muslim, or Hindu family (among many other possibilities). I'm sure I would still have felt the same compelling need to identify and know God. In those situations, I might have called Him by another name but He would still be God. I would likely have felt just as convinced that my religion was just as "right" as Christianity has been for me here. In either case, I firmly believe God would have accepted me and provided the same guidance and help as He has for me here.

I hold a variety of beliefs regarding social issues that might cause some to label me as a "liberal" and might even cause them to question the legitimacy of my faith. I recall thinking that way earlier in my life when I was sure I knew everything. I viewed things in black and white then and was sure that a "real" Christian would believe and act and vote in certain ways. I don't view the world that way anymore. I've made peace with ambiguity and am comfortable acknowledging that I see most issues in shades of gray these days. I am aware that this may annoy or offend some who read this. This is not my intention. But it may be an unavoidable consequence. I am quite willing to agree to disagree. But I am aware that some others are not okay with this. Ultimately that is their issue, not mine.

Religious Versus Spiritual

There is a difference between hope in and hope for. Hope in implies that hope is drawn from a type of external power source such as God, religion or philosophical beliefs. Hope for generally refers to things we hope will happen. They may or may not be connected to the One we hope in.

Historically the terms religious and spiritual meant the same things. But over time they became somewhat disconnected. These days an estimated twenty percent of Americans describe themselves as spiritual but not religious (SBNR). So what is the difference? Perhaps we should start by identifying what is the same, namely a belief in some form of a Higher Power.[2]

Religious

Those who are religious believe in God or a set of gods and some form of organized religion. A study of 346 people from a wide range of religious backgrounds indicated they associated religion with higher levels of church attendance and commitment to traditional beliefs. They typically followed the rules, rituals and practices of said religion.[3] In the US the majority of such people claim Christianity as their religion but numerous other religions are represented as well. The term religious has come to have both positive and negative meanings. It has a positive meaning for persons who find their religion to be deeply meaningful and who gain value in the associated practices.

Others sometimes use the term religious to describe someone who makes a show of their beliefs to impress others but does not appear to "practice what they preach." An example is a person said to be a Sunday Christian meaning he pretends to be religious on Sundays but fails to demonstrate the same belief system the other six days of the week. In other words, he is thought to be a hypocrite or a fraud. Worse yet, there are those who profess religious beliefs but use their position within the church to manipulate and deceive others for their own personal gain. In my opinion, these are all frauds and I've learned to avoid them whenever possible.

Spirituality

A person's spirituality is more authentic in my opinion than most religious rituals. Yet I am also aware that for some, participation in certain religious rituals can be deeply meaningful and may serve to enrich their spiritual experience. It is very individual. It can also be a valuable resource for coping with cancer, and has been shown to actually extend life.[4] The National Cancer Institute defines spirituality as one's belief about the meaning of life. Such beliefs may be expressed through religious practices, the arts, communing with nature, meditation, yoga, prayer, or other means.

Those who identify themselves as spiritual but not religious (SBNR) often reject traditional organized religion. Many have had negative experiences with churches or church leaders. For example, they may have perceived church leaders as being more concerned with big building projects and promoting the organization rather than promoting spirituality. Worse, they may have come to view them as closed-minded hypocrites. Some may have even experienced manipulation and emotional, financial, or sexual abuse from leadership.[5] Needless to say, this may have left them feeling disconnected, untrusting, and angry toward organized religion.

In the same study as mentioned above, some in the SBNR group were more interested in mysticism and non-traditional beliefs and practices. Some were more likely to be agnostic and to pick from a wide range of alternative religious philosophies. They were less likely to be involved in traditional forms of worship. They typically view spirituality as a journey closely connected with the pursuit of personal growth.[6]

Those who identify as SBNR may claim a form of belief based upon variations of one or more religions (Buddhism, Hinduism, Christianity, etc.). Further they often describe a connection to a larger reality such as the human race, nature, or the universe.[7]

A New Group?

In my own experience I have met a number of people who profess to be spiritual but not religious Christians. So I suppose their acronym might be SBNRC? In most cases they profess belief in God and Jesus but view the bible as a spiritually inspired written work rather than the literal word of God as described by most conservative

Christians. In addition, many believe in greater freedom of expression and thought and are described as having more liberal beliefs than their conservative counterparts. In spite of this, they still view themselves as devoted Christians. For example, many years ago I became friends with Gina, another nurse where I worked. During our many discussions I learned that she was not married but had lived with her significant other for fifteen years. They were deeply committed to one another and had a loving and respectful relationship. Furthermore, I learned that she believed gays and lesbians were as likely as anyone else to go to heaven. The most interesting thing to me was that she considered herself a Christian and had a very active prayer life.

I had come from the experience of living and socializing among a very conservative Christian population where a person like my friend Gina would have been quickly judged as being out of God's will. If she did not respond to "counseling" and change her ways she might well have been ostracized from the group. The Christians in that world viewed everything in black and white but my new friend, whom I deeply respected and liked, viewed things in shades of gray. This experience challenged me to rethink some of my own beliefs because I realized that Gina was more authentic than half the "Christians" I knew; more authentic than I was. She would easily have fit into the SBNRC group. And I've come to see myself there as well.

Belief in an Afterlife

Whether individuals believe in an afterlife and how they describe it varies widely. Major factors influencing such beliefs include specific religious affiliation and family influences during upbringing. Most Christians believe in some variation of heaven and, slightly less commonly, variations of hell. They generally believe that after death they will enter one or the other depending upon various factors. Most significant among these are acceptance of Jesus as their savior, forgiveness of sins, and having lived a good life which included love and concern for others.

Atheists, Agnostics, and Hope

The concept of hope is closely tied to religious or spiritual beliefs for those who claim them. This makes sense given the fact that most people find a sense of purpose or meaning that is dictated or influenced by their chosen religion or spiritual traditions. In fact, for most believers, the two are so closely tied together that they question the ability of nonbelievers to feel and maintain real hope, especially as related to death and dying.

So what about those who profess no belief in God or an afterlife? Can they still experience hope? Believers may be doubtful, but nonbelievers say, "yes." Many people who are atheistic (believe in no God or gods) or agnostic (question the reality of God or gods) indicate they feel great hope, even though it may be fueled by a different set of beliefs.[8]

Others may feel challenged to understand this. But I believe everyone is entitled to the same respect regardless what their belief system might be. When someone says they find something deeply meaningful and are inspired to feel hopeful, who am I to argue? Faith and belief are subjective and don't lend themselves to observation or measurement by others. They must simply be taken on faith.

Some twenty years ago I was making regular three-hour road trips to graduate school. For part of that time, I carpooled with a good friend of mine. With a three-hour drive each way we had plenty of time to talk. In doing so, we touched on a variety of topics and as good friends who deeply respected one another, we had the rare luxury of being able to disagree in ways that were challenging and insightful but not hurtful. One day when we happened upon the topic of religion my friend stated that as an atheist she had no belief whatsoever in God. I paused briefly and then surprised us both by saying, "Wow, you must have an enormous amount of faith." She gave me an odd, questioning look and then repeated herself. "No Sharon, I don't believe in God at all." She thought I had either misunderstood her or was making fun. In fact, it was neither. It simply occurred to me, as I explained to her, that it must take a huge amount of faith to believe in nothing, no God, no Creator, no superpower of any kind. I said that to me, God just made sense. Without Him I had a difficult time coming up with a better explanation for creation, the meaning of life, why we are all here, and so on. She then paused and said "Huh. I never thought of it like that." It didn't occur to me at the time, to ask her what inspired her to feel hopeful. I wish I had.

So lately I've been wondering what sort of things might inspire hope in the person who is agnostic or atheistic. I've discovered several answers. Some express hope in their fellow human beings, in a belief that the human race is evolving and will eventually overcome obstacles like injustice, racial discrimination, and famine.[9] Many are inspired by the inherent goodness of people; demonstrated by how their best qualities seem to rise to the surface when circumstances are at their worst. For example, think about the many times when people who may not even know one another join together to overcome adversity to achieve a common goal. The passengers on United Airlines flight 93 unified under the direst of circumstances to resist terrorists and force the airplane off its deadly course. In doing so they saved hundreds of lives of people unknown to them; all the while knowing their own lives would be forfeited. At the same time many others put themselves in harm's way and entered the World Trade Center towers in the hope of saving others. Upon entering the buildings, many knew they might never escape. Three hundred and forty-three firefighters and sixty law enforcement officers sacrificed their own lives in an attempt to save those in the world trade center towers.[10] Other examples abound and are too numerous to describe. Many who sacrificed themselves were persons of faith. Some were not. In either case they believed in something greater than themselves and acted accordingly.

Now let's consider the agnostic or atheistic person who is facing a terminal illness. Do they have reason to hope? I confess that I myself have sometimes wondered how they could. Being a person of faith, I cannot imagine walking the path I am on without the love, support and help I believe comes from God. After having pondered this topic for some time, I have come to realize that my hope is both a hope in and a hope for. Theirs may be primarily a hope for although I'm sure it varies with each individual and I'm in no place to judge. In any case I expect that we all hope for many of the same things. After all, when death draws near, don't we all hope for some semblance of the following?

- Hope for loved ones to draw near.

- Hope for reconciliation with certain persons in our lives.

- Hope for pain relief.

- Hope for caregivers who listen, acknowledge our needs and provide a caring response.

- Hope for a peaceful death.

- Hope for a dignified death.

- Hope for freedom from fear and anxiety.

- Hope for meaning and purpose.

Dr. Jerome Groopman wrote "The Anatomy of Hope," an insightful book that looks at how people prevail in the face of severe illness. He describes his father, an agnostic, as very doubtful about an afterlife. Yet he also describes him as extremely hopeful and looking to love as the force that would shape his family's future. After his death he expected the power of memory to keep his presence alive for his family.[11] Is this not also a form of hope?

Spirituality

Spirituality is about seeking and enhancing a connection with our creator, with the universe, with nature, and even with other human beings. When we hurt others, we damage this connection. But when we are empathetic and helpful to others, I believe we enrich it. If we damage nature, abuse the resources of our planet, or simply take it and our amazing universe for granted, I believe we impair this connection. Yet we can enhance it through our appreciation of nature and taking measures to protect our planet and the resources it offers. The universe is vast and overwhelming, beautiful and mysterious. Each time I learn something more about it I am reminded of the power and creativity of my God. But if we fail to seek and nurture a relationship with our creator I believe we rob ourselves of an amazing, life-changing opportunity for spiritual growth and understanding.

Upon death I do not believe we cease to exist. This notion simply makes no logical sense to me. I recall learning in my chemistry classes that energy never ceases to exist. It simply changes forms. What are we if not a remarkable form of energy? When we die I believe we simply change form and experience a change of location. It may be lightyears away or might be right here, in another dimension. Either way, our spiritual selves exit our physical bodies and continue to exist in that form.

This belief is confirmed by the millions of people who have had near death experiences (NDEs). One such person described dying to be as "simple as walking into the next room."[12] Many also believe that we eventually return to the earth in physical form through reincarnation. The purpose, as I understand it, is to take another turn in the classroom of life where we continue to learn and grow in ways not possible when we are in spirit. I believe I will eventually learn the truth of the matter and will have the opportunity to question God about it if I wish.

I am puzzled by organizations or people who think they have God all figured out. How can this be possible when He is so infinite, so mysterious and so much larger than our small minds could ever fully grasp? To ever think we can fully know and understand God seems rather arrogant to me. The only one who really knows the complete truth is God Himself. The rest of us are bumbling along through life, doing the best we can and most of us make plenty of mistakes along the way. We are all fallible and none of us knows the entire truth. For this reason, we need to humble ourselves and extend one another a great deal of grace.

Prayer

There's an old saying "There are no atheists in fox holes." This refers to soldiers in time of war who are trapped under fire. Whether they claim to believe in God or not, they usually find themselves reaching out in prayer, seeking help from God or some other unnamed source. After all, what is prayer but hope in action? When we feel threatened by danger, it seems a normal human reaction to seek some form of help and comfort.

There are many types of prayer and they are not always spoken to God. Some pray to other religious figures including Jesus, Mohammed, Buddha, the Virgin Mary, or numerous saints. Yet in all cases prayer is a way of seeking contact with someone or something greater than ourselves. And in most cases it involves asking for help or guidance.

Nouwen describes prayer as the manifestation of hope and expectation of new things.[13] He further describes the difference between prayers of "little faith" and prayers of "real hope." Prayers of little hope generally include a list of the items we want or the outcomes we wish for.[14] Author Kathleen Norris calls these the simple "gimme, gimme" prayers.[15] Nouwen points out these types of prayers are often based on fear and anxiety and we view tangible results (or lack thereof) as proof that our hope was well-founded (or not).[16]

An example might be if I pray for a new car. Then if I receive the car, my hope and faith would seem to have been well-founded and God has answered my request. But what if the opposite happens? If I don't get the new car, then is the failure God's or mine? Was my faith too weak? Did God not hear me? Is He withholding the car from me? Am I being punished for something? Many seem to view faith in this way. This form of belief system seems shallow to me because it is generally focused on the immediate future and often on material things.

Journal August 2010
Prayer

Norris suggests that the opposite of hope is fear and despair.[17] I would tend to agree since I can feel the difference when my prayers are based in fear versus hope and faith. Faith fuels hope and hope fuels faith. They both are grounded in trust. Fear feeds despair and hopelessness. I know which of these I prefer but all too often I find myself praying the prayers of fear. I'm trying to become more conscious of this so I can make the shift to faith/trust/hope-based prayers.

"Lord please help me pray from a place of hope and faith,

since I know that you see the big picture and you seek the greater good. Help me let gear and keep my heart, mind, and hands open to You."

I read a section from Amazing Grace this morning and was deeply touched as I felt God confirming much of what I believed He had been telling me since this odyssey began. The author discusses the difference between those who pray regularly with serious intent, and those who pray superficial prayers where they merely ask for items on their wish list. The former is based on a deep sense of gratitude for everything they've been given, including their problems.[18] I recognized that the pattern of my past prayers were mostly of the "gimme, gimme" variety. But I want my communication and my entire relationship with God to become deeper and more meaningful than that.

When we pray we most often focus on the immediate future. We want something or someone in our lives to be different. So we ask God to fix the situation or change the person. What we so often forget is that our vision is extremely poor. We see only the immediate situation and even then are prone to flawed perception. Our ideas about how the future should look are even less accurate. For us to dictate to God how it ought to be is absurd. Better for us to trust that He sees the big picture and knows far better than we do, what the long term goals are. This concept is pointed out nicely in I Corinthians 13:12 which states, "For now we see only a reflection as in a mirror; then we shall see face to face. Now I know in part; then I shall know fully, even as I am fully known (NIV)."

I appreciate this scripture because it points out how flawed our vision is now. The implication, then, is that our prayers may be flawed as well, especially when we ask for specific items and specific, detailed outcomes. On the other hand, God's vision is perfect.

He sees the present and the distant future in accurate detail. Once we are with Him, our vision will be perfected as well. We will finally see things clearly and understand all. Consequently, when I am unsure how to pray, I make my prayers more general. I pray for God's will to be done. I also pray for things like guidance, learning, wisdom, and spiritual growth for myself and others.

JOURNAL AUGUST 2010
THE BIG PICTURE

I recall once reading a Facebook post which said that people with cancer only ever wished for one thing; to be cured. I'm sure the author's intent was good but I found myself in disagreement. There are many things more important than my healing; like learning, growing, helping others, and fulfilling God's purpose for my life.

Eventually we will all die. So what is the point of only ever praying for healing? Sometimes God has other plans. Norris describes situations in which the best we can do is to pray for God's mercy; asking for a quick, peaceful death. She further explains that instead of asking for what we want, perhaps we should ask God what He wants of us, letting Him change us and make us more grateful for what we've already been given.[19]

So rather than demanding a cure, I've found greater peace of mind in praying for mercy; to make my passing peaceful, and free of pain, fear, or anxiety. I have also asked for "more time" without specifying how much time that should be. It seemed arrogant of me to dictate to God how long I should live. But I did ask for "more time" to see my unborn grandchildren and to be with family. The details are up to Him.

Will He honor my requests? So far He seems to be, since I'm still here. But regardless, I've noticed that I feel a much greater sense of honesty and comfort in this sort of prayer than in demanding healing.

God rarely answers prayers in the manner we expect. Yet He always answers them. Sometimes the answer is "no" or "not now." But usually it is simply different than anything we envision. This may not be obvious at first, but with time, faith, and trust we can see it, but only if we keep our eyes open.

I realized one day, long ago, that I rarely took the time or had the awareness to thank God for His many answers to prayer. So I challenged myself at that time to become more consistently aware so that I would be more likely to notice such things. Over time it happened. When I prayed, I made a mental note to "stay tuned" so that I would consciously notice when the answer appeared. Then when it did, I made sure to consciously express my gratitude.

The Key

As I considered my most common prayers, I felt foolish that I would be so selfish and small-minded as to waste God's precious time and attention on my small issues. Yet as I pondered it I felt God pointing out to me that as a parent He takes great joy in doing things for His children, as human parents do for our children. In fact, the smaller and sillier the issue or item, the more fun He might have in taking care of it for us.

As a mother of three, I could relate to this. I thought about how much I enjoy doing things for my children. Sometimes the smallest things can bring the most joy as they realize that I did it "just because," out of love. Not because I had to or even because they needed it, but because I wanted to and I knew it would bless them.

As I pondered the subject God pointed out to me that He feels the same way about us. I had never envisioned Him this way. In my earlier life I saw Him as the all-powerful, judgmental, often angry, and nearly always impersonal God who was frequently displeased at my failures. Consequently, I virtually always felt guilty and inadequate. For the first time in my life, I now saw him differently. I slowly began to realize that he is a loving, attentive, humorous, fun-loving father who wanted a close relationship with me, his daughter. Having my own children, helped me to understand this. This transformation in our relationship didn't happen quickly but it did happen. The first time I specifically recall a close interaction of this sort, I was at work. I needed to prepare the nursing lab for the next day. But I couldn't find the key to one of the supply cabinets. It had been months since I'd been in the cabinet and I had no memory of what had become of the key. As I searched throughout the many cabinets in several rooms I felt my frustration begin to rise. Then I heard His small voice in the back of my mind say, "Ask me." It stopped me in my tracks. I hesitated because it seemed such a silly, small thing to pray about. It certainly didn't match up to big problems like world hunger or the Middle-East conflict. But He did tell me to ask. So I thought, "Why not?" I had nothing to lose. So I said a quick, simple prayer in which I asked Him to please help me locate the key. Almost immediately an image came into my mind of a key on top of a specific cabinet (one of many) far above my eye level. It can't be that simple, I thought. But I had to know, so I pushed a chair up to the cabinet in question and climbed on it. The top was still out of my sight but at least I could now reach it. I extended my arm up to the cabinet top and placed my hand right on top of a dusty key. I was surprised, amazed, and as pleased as I could possibly have been. I laughed out loud as I thanked God for his faithfulness, even in such a tiny, insignificant matter. Of course He knew it wasn't tiny to me. It was actually huge to me, and it marked the beginning of an entirely new relationship between us.

Since that day I've been more consistent in asking for help, even with the little things and then staying tuned to note if and when an answer manifests itself. The amazing thing is that I came to realize that God always answered. I can't tell you how many times He has helped me locate my keys, glasses, important papers, and even something as silly as the TV remote. Always, though not always right away. But only when I remembered to ask. Even more important is that I began talking to Him on a daily basis. I say talking rather than praying because so often that's what it felt like. A personal on-going conversation. As a result, I've felt my relationship with him deepen in a spiritually relaxed manner; less religious (to my way of thinking) and certainly more real.

Faith

It's one thing to trust God with the little things, and the process described above helped me to do this. It's another, or seems so, to trust Him with the big things, like the mountain of debt I had acquired, my children's lives, and cancer. But I think God was preparing me. He knew the cancer would come up later in my life, so I think He was teaching me about trust, first using the little things. And as time went by, with larger and larger things. In truth, I've come to realize that it's all the same. It may feel like little things versus big things. But God is equally able to take care of it all. It was just my faith that needed to grow and God knew I would be more successful starting with the "small" stuff.

Ms. Norris notes how for most people faith seems to fluctuate, feeling stronger on some days, weaker on others.[20] Yet she understands the value in paying attention which allows us to notice God's faithfulness to us. Over time, this prompts our faith and hope to grow.

As I've pondered God's message to me to trust in Him I've wondered if trust and faith are the same. I think they must be or are closely related. In fact, I suspect that trust may be faith in action.

I've wrestled with my own stance in regard to what God's will might be for me and how I am to pray and to believe. There are other people who immediately (and it seemed to me, with little thought) decided that God would heal me. As I've chatted with them it became obvious they were reluctant to discuss any other possibilities. This is interesting to me given that it is my body and my life in question. Why is considering the possibility that I may die so terrifying to them? In many cases they have nicely, but rather abruptly, shut me down. I get the impression that they are frightened by the prospect that I might die and seem to think that even allowing their mind to consider the possibility would be a betrayal of their own faith. I understand that there are also elements of love and concern for me that are a dimension of this response. I appreciate this. But there is something more at play here and that is what I'm referring to. It reminds me of some of the religious doctrine of churches I've attended in past years—and one of many reasons I stopped attending for a time. There seemed to be a belief that intelligent thought, questioning God, and considering possibilities other than those sanctioned by the church are diametrically opposed to having faith. As if I simply refuse to let my mind consider any other option, then God has no choice but to do what I've set my mind on and, in this case, heal me. There seems to be a strong belief that this mindset constitutes faith. I don't think I believe that any more. I'm not sure I ever did—it was just one of many annoying belief systems of the churches I attended that used to drive me nuts. It seemed to imply that if God would just conform to our rules then all would be well. If we only let our minds dwell on what we want to have happen then God has no choice but to respond accordingly. Is this absurd or what?

Since my odyssey began, the messages I believe I've heard from God have been Trust Me and Be Grateful. This is still what I am hearing. As a result, I've pondered both notions quite a lot. I haven't heard God say for certain that He is going to heal me. I haven't heard Him say that He is not going to heal me either. At first I thought the failure was mine—that if I could just hear Him more clearly I would know. Now I've come to believe that this is intentional on His part. He's not saying either way. In any case, as I have pondered the whole notion of trust, it occurred to me that being uncertain of the outcome puts me in a position where I have the opportunity to walk in faith and learn more about what trust really means. For if I had an ironclad guarantee from God that I will eventually be healed, where would be the need for faith?

And if I had everything in my life that I had ever wanted and if everything were perfect then would I feel grateful or would I simply take it all for granted? I've noticed that the absence of the thing I want nearly always helps me to appreciate it far more when it manifests. For example:

- Pain causes me to appreciate comfort.

- Ugliness causes me to appreciate beauty.

- Debt causes me to appreciate abundance.

- Fatigue causes me to appreciate rest.

- Hunger causes me to appreciate a full belly.

- Fear causes me to appreciate peace of mind.

And so on . . .

God knows this about me. I think He knows this is true about most people. So He creates or allows experiences that help us learn gratitude, faith, and the many other lessons we are to learn in this life.

I believe we humans are generally confused about our purpose here on planet Earth. We think we are here to have fun, accumulate things, make money, and live a happily-ever-after, stress-free life of comfort and abundance. We may periodically do any or all of these things and sometimes they may be blessings from God. But they are not necessarily "rewards" for good behavior and their absence isn't necessarily "punishment" for bad behavior. It's all about the process of learning whatever lessons we must learn: trust, faith, gratitude, love, generosity, humility . . . the lessons are probably countless. I think this is much of why we are here. It's not about accumulating money or stuff. If it were, then I suspect God would have made some provision for us being able to take these things with us when we die. But we cannot. We take nothing physical. We are only allowed to take non-physical things like love, faith, gratitude, and wisdom.

Essence of Faith

"So we fix our eyes, not on what is seen, but on what is unseen, since what is seen is temporary, but what is unseen is eternal." Second Corinthians 4:18

I like this verse because it captures at least a part of the essence of faith which is a challenging notion to define. For those who claim it faith is real, powerful and sometimes even lifesaving. But trying to describe faith to one who requires objective (visible, measurable) evidence can feel impossible. I love what Norris has to say on the matter. She describes faith as a fluctuating sort of "energy" that requires us to pay attention and keep our eyes open.[21]

∽

It's an odd thing to find myself praying that God will spare me from many of the very things my patients have gone through. I've seen enough to be fearful of the possibilities. Being a nurse isn't always a good thing. But then I think, "What makes me so special? Why should God spare me from the things that so many others have suffered?" The answer to the first question is simple: I am no more or less special than any of them. God loved them. He loves me.

The answer to the second question is less clear. I know that each person's situation and purpose is unique. I don't know that God will spare me from suffering. But I know that He can. So my prayers take on two forms. First that He will be merciful and spare me whenever possible. Secondly that He will help me to bear whatever I must and help me trust in His higher purpose. The path is unpredictable and largely unknown. I feel as though I'm walking nearly blind, unable to see the twists, turns and obstacles that lay before me. The outcome, however, seems certain. Each day God illuminates the path just enough for me to take each baby step. He does this in many ways; some obvious, some so subtle as to be nearly imperceptible. I wish it were always clear and certain. I wish I could always feel sure of myself, sure about what I'm supposed to do. But then, where would be the need for faith?

Chapter 5

1. Isaiah 40:31 *The Holy Bible, New International Version.* Zondervan Publishing House, Grand Rapids, 1984.

2. Robert C. Fuller. "Spiritual, But Not Religious." www.beliefnet.com/Entertainment/Books/2002/07/Spiritual-But-Not-Religious.aspx#67HfKSCMWXL1L879.99 (accessed 3/29/2017).

3. Ibid

4. Very Well, https://www.verywell.com/lung-cancer-and-spirituality-2249240 (accessed 3/29/2017).

5. American Atheist: https://www.atheists.org/activism/resources/about-atheism/ (accessed 3/29/2017).

6. Ibid

7. Ibid

8. Atheist Foundation of Australia Inc. "Frequently Asked Questions," atheistfoundation.org.au (accessed 11/2/2015).

9. Ibid

10. 9/11 by the Numbers Death, destruction, charity, salvation, war, money, real estate, spouses, babies, and other September 11 statistics. http://nymag.com/news/articles/wtc/1year/numbers.htm

11. Groopman, Ibid. Kindle location 1693.

12. Helen Keller, Brainy Quotes, copyright 2001-2017, https://www.brainyquote.com/quotes/quotes/h/helenkelle117408.html (accessed 3/29/2017)

13. Nouwen Ibid. p 63, 68.

14. Ibid. 68-71.

15. Kathleen Norris. *Amazing Grace: A Vocabulary of Faith.* Riverhead books, New York, 1998. p. 60.

16. Nouwen p. 68-69.

17. Norris, Ibid, p. 181.

18. Ibid, p. 60.

19. Ibid.

20. Ibid. 170.

21. Ibid. 169.

Chapter 6:
Hope Versus Realism

"Our generation is realistic, for we have come to know man as he really is. After all, man is that being who invented the gas chambers of Auschwitz; however, he is also that being who entered those gas chambers upright, with the Lord's Prayer or the Shema Yisrael on his lips." [1]

Maintaining a balanced state of hope versus realism is a continual challenge. Being optimistic feels easy when all is going well. It takes little effort and is certainly where I prefer to be. Most of us have a tendency to hear and interpret facts in a biased manner to keep ourselves there. An old example is to view the glass as half full rather than half empty. But as soon as challenges arise we may be knocked off balance before we know what hit us. Depending on the nature of the challenge we may experience it as a small "bump in the road" or a major life crisis.

Selective Hearing

When I worked in the ICU, I often found myself challenged to answer certain questions from my patients' family members. If the prognosis was good, it was fairly easy to do. But when the prognosis was grim it was much more difficult. I wanted to be honest and in certain cases begin preparing them for a bad outcome. I did not want to encourage false hope but neither did I wish to destroy all hope. I also knew from experience they were prone to "selective hearing" and would generally focus only on what they perceived to be positive news. It seemed that no matter how careful I was in wording my answers, family members only heard what they were ready to hear. Furthermore, since most families were not familiar with the medical world, they would focus on the simple things they understood, such as basic vital signs and simple nutrition issues. But in the ICU, situations are rarely that simple. Vital signs may look good, and it might be because the patient is truly doing well and is on the mend. Or it might be due to the vasoactive drugs being pumped into him, the ventilator that is breathing for him, and a cooling blanket that has dropped his body temperature from 105°F to normal. In the first case, the body is maintaining everything on its own. In the second case it's not and without the extra measures provided by nursing care, the patient would most likely be dead or dying. In the ICU, basic vital signs may be among the last numbers to fail. But if the observer is unable to interpret the whole picture, he will not realize this. So the hopeful family member often looks at semi-normal vital signs and believes their loved one is getting better. It's up to nurses and physicians to interpret things for them, but we do so while walking a tightrope between hope and realism.

Dual Role of Nurse and Younger Sister

This story is an example from my own life, of the thorny path walked by health care providers and patients' loved ones as everyone tries to maintain hope in the face of extreme odds (realism). In this story I found myself playing a dual role as the patient's younger sister who also happened to be a nurse. Throughout the experience I felt extremely torn between reality (as I saw it) and the need for my family to cling to hope. As the little sister I also needed to hope that my big brother could recover and I wanted to encourage my family without feeding false hope. Yet from the outset, the situation was so dire that I seriously doubted he would or could ever recover. In fact, it seemed hopeless. This created an extreme dilemma for me. How honest should I be? If I told them what I really thought, I feared I would destroy their hopes. I didn't want that to happen and I wasn't sure if I even had the right. We all needed hope. And though true miracles seem to be rare, we all believed that one could happen for Rob if God willed it. So there I was, caught between being the little sister and being the ICU nurse. To some degree my family recognized my dilemma and encouraged me to "stop being a nurse" for that time and "just be the sister." I appreciated their intent but I had no idea how to do so. I had entered nursing school in 1987 and had been a nurse ever since. It wasn't just a job; it had become a central part of my identity. I could no more stop thinking like a nurse than I could stop breathing. So I mostly kept my true thoughts to myself while trying to be helpful in playing the role of medical translator and little sister. This story is based on my point of view and is largely reconstructed from the daily emails I wrote at the time, to distant family and friends.

Robbin

My oldest brother Robbin died on November 24, 2009, six months before I was diagnosed with cancer. He was fifty-eight years old and other than being overweight, was quite healthy at the time he contracted the H1N1 influenza.

Rob had always been something of a loner, choosing not to marry and living alone (with his cats) in Portland, Oregon, some distance from the rest of us. In earlier years I believe this had to do with the fact that he was an alcoholic and was still wrestling with demons from his youth. Exactly what they were, I could only guess. He never discussed them. But our family, or more specifically our father and his family had enough dysfunction for a hundred families, so it could have been anything. For many years Rob lived a life of seclusion, rarely reaching out or responding to anyone else except for our mother. As her firstborn son, mom loved him more than anything and worried about him and his solitary life. She never gave up on him. She sent him letters and cards and sewed things for him and his tiny trailer home. On several occasions, with his consent, she drove her own tiny motor home to Portland and became one of his neighbors for a time in the trailer court in which he lived. They worked out a system by mutual agreement where Rob would leave his curtains open when he was up for company and keep them closed when he wasn't. Over time, Mom became familiar with the small but meaningful life Rob had created for himself. Around the outside of his trailer were dozens of pots and planters in which he grew and tended a tiny garden. He loved growing things and loved to cook, so gardening seemed a natural hobby for him, even though he lacked any real ground space to do it. Rob never married, nor had any children that we knew of. But within the trailer court there were a number of children each with their own dysfunctional families and their own stories. Over time they came to realize that although Rob might give the appearance of a grumpy old man, he was actually a teddy bear at heart. As time passed, they developed a certain friendship where the kids felt free to bring their broken bikes to Rob to see if he could fix them. The last ten years of his life, he worked in a high end mountain bicycle shop, so he had the knowledge and skills to do this. Besides fixing things, he took his role of "uncle Rob" seriously and looked out for the children in the court. There were days when his curtains were drawn and the kids knew not to knock on his door. But other days when the curtains were open and Rob was tending his garden or sitting on his porch step, they knew they could approach him and get help with their broken bikes and, sometimes, with their broken lives. Rob rarely interfered in their family lives but he had a way of instilling confidence in the children and letting them know that they could trust in him as well as in themselves.

Mom's presence was therapeutic for Rob. She respected his privacy but spent quality time with him whenever she could. She would sew and mend things for him and subtly but consistently send him the message that she believed in him. They often joined one another for dinner in one of their tiny homes and enjoyed a one-on-one relationship that they hadn't had time for since he was very young. Rob was the oldest of six children, so his childhood was a busy, hectic one. I think he loved this special time when he had Mom all to himself. That her presence made a difference became obvious the day he told her that he had decided to join AA. From that day on, there was no more alcohol in his home. Since he wasn't spending money on booze, for the first time in his adult life, he was able to save for other things. It was so rewarding to see him take pleasure and a certain amount of pride in the things he was able to earn and enjoy. Examples included a television, a computer, and eventually a used car. This was the first car he had owned in many, many years.

Rob was a homebody and rarely traveled. Since he stopped drinking he became more social than before and welcomed visits from family passing through Portland. He was quite frugal with his money and rarely, if ever, ate out. But our sister, Stephenie, and her family knew that it was a special treat for him to eat a meal in a restaurant while catching up on family news. So when they were in town they always made a special point of taking him to dinner. Steph often compares him to a little kid on Christmas day on those occasions. He took such great joy in the luxury of eating out and special time with family.

Robbin also became known for infrequent, but lengthy and chatty phone calls to his siblings. Knowing this, I bought him phone cards for Christmas, on several occasions. The first time he called me the first words out of his mouth were "I got minutes for Christmas!! I got lots of minutes! So I'm gonna use 'em!"

Rob eventually got rid of his trailer (which was starting to fall apart) and rented a little one-bedroom duplex apartment on Suave Island located just outside of Portland in the Columbia River. The island looked like something out of a storybook. Lush green fields, rolling farmland, acres of vineyards, and an open-air farmers market. I'm sure it was Rob's idea of heaven and reminded him of the Willamette Valley where we had all grown up together. We couldn't have been happier for him and knew it was a blessed change from the crime-filled neighborhood where he had lived for so many years.

November 2009

When tragedy strikes we rarely get any sort of warning. It was a typical Monday and we were all busy with our various jobs when I learned the local police had knocked on Mom's door that afternoon with the news that Rob had been admitted to Kaiser Permanente hospital in Portland. All the police knew was that he was on a ventilator in the ICU. This left me with my stomach in knots. I knew being on a ventilator meant he was in real trouble. We were to eventually learn that he'd had the flu for a week before seeing a doctor for difficulty breathing. The flu had attacked his lungs causing pneumonia and by the time he sought medical care he was deathly ill.

Over the next several hours I managed to get faculty coverage for my various duties, and packed a suitcase and met up with the rest of my family. We quickly shared information and made travel plans to Portland. Before hitting the road my brother called the hospital and spoke with Rob's nurse. As I stood by listening to his side of the conversation, I felt anxious to ask her some "nurse" questions which might clue me in to his real condition. Once I got the phone I fired off specific questions about the vent settings and felt my heart sink as she provided answers. Rob had developed a complication known as acute respiratory distress syndrome (ARDS) which had a very high mortality rate. They had set the ventilator to maximize efforts to get oxygen into his blood, but it wasn't working very well. I knew right then that his chances of survival were extremely slim. I suddenly wasn't so glad to be the family nurse. How could I explain to the rest of my family the gravity of Rob's condition without robbing them of hope? And that was to be the ongoing question over the next ten days, as I became the family letter-writer and sent daily updates to other relatives. My e-mails to them tells most of the rest of the story. The first one (below) was written after our first day at the hospital.

November 17, 2009

Rob is critically ill and as his nurse said this evening "doesn't have any reserves" so he has a real fight on his hands. We spent all day at the hospital and as much time at his side as they would allow. Everyone has been kind and supportive; including security personnel who helped us find our way around at one this morning. It's comforting to know that he has been in good hands since they were unable to track down family for a couple of days.

As I feared, Rob is in ARDS. His numbers have improved slightly today but his doctor only gives him a fifty-fifty chance of survival, which is actually better than I expected.

They started him on an experimental drug for the H1N1 flu virus since responses with Tamiflu haven't been very good.

It's hard being the sister. I much prefer being the nurse where I feel a greater sense of control and am probably not aware of how much is at stake. I'm used to watching the family dynamics come into play. But it's weird and it's painful being a part of the family as I also maintain the nurse's perspective.

NOVEMBER 20, 2009

What a wild ride it's been, but not a fun one. There are more details than I could possibly remember but I'll try to summarize. Rob's condition has deteriorated. Lab results indicate his kidneys are beginning to fail. Each time I enter his room I can't help but read the story being told by all the equipment. His ventilator settings scream desperation. One of the IV fluids battles to maintain a failing blood pressure. His plummeting oxygen saturation level tells the scariest story of all. It speaks of the oxygen that isn't making it into his blood. When blood is starved for oxygen, so is everything else. His heart, lungs, kidneys, liver, and brain are all suffocating. How much of this can he handle and still survive?

After much deliberation my family decided to opt for a treatment that might give him a chance. ECMO (extracorporeal membrane oxygenation) is a high tech machine used to remove blood (similar to a heart-lung bypass machine), oxygenate it, and then return it to the body. Only two hospitals on the West Coast offer it. Fortunately for Rob, one of them is here in Portland, but at another hospital. So he must be moved and I wonder if he can handle it. The ECMO will be a last-ditch effort.

Rob's heart keeps going into atrial fibrillation, an abnormal rhythm. This bought him another piece of equipment; an external cardioverter with patches in place so they can cardiovert (shock) him as needed. This has occurred many times, three while my mom, younger brother (Roger), and I were in the room. Each time they shocked his heart I felt my own heart breaking. By 6 a.m. a large medical team arrived to prepare Rob for the ECMO and hospital transfer.

Unfortunately, it became much more traumatic than necessary because of a huge communication SNAFU. We had already discussed the issue at length and decided that we did not want Rob treated for any lethal heart arrhythmias. If his heart were to stop as a result, then so be it. This seemed the closest we could come to agreeing on anything near a "no code" status. This information had not been relayed to the ECMO team. And the ECMO team failed to tell us that heart arrhythmias were so common with the initiation of ECMO that they were viewed as nearly normal. In addition, they did not make it clear to us that the ECMO would be initiated before transfer. Apparently patients tolerate the stress of transfer better with ECMO already in place. It makes sense to me now but I didn't know it then.

So my family and I were returning from the cafeteria early this morning just in time to find the ECMO team in place, coding Rob. One nurse was straddling him, administering CPR while the rest of the team stood around his bed pushing various medications and preparing to transfer him. We became upset because we thought they were going against our expressed wishes. Some of us began yelling for them to stop while my most analytical brother wanted to ask questions and have a discussion. It was total chaos. At that point the physician who led the team pulled us aside and clarified what was going on from his perspective. He also apologized for not having explained things more clearly ahead of time. By this time, Rob's heart rhythm had been restored to normal and so we agreed to proceed.

Lessons learned: Just because family members think they've agreed on a plan doesn't mean it gets correctly communicated to the critical members of the healthcare team or that someone won't have last-minute questions.

So now Rob is in the ICU of a different hospital, Emanuel Legacy. It has a different atmosphere and much stricter visitation rules. It is taking some adjustment on our part but we are adapting by remembering that it is all about Rob and not us. It also helped that the staff at the other hospital was so incredibly flexible and supportive and allowed us to spend a great deal of time with him. It gave us each the chance to say what was in our hearts, so at least if it ends for him now, we won't feel cheated of that opportunity.

Doctors have warned us that he may never fully recover (to pre-illness health) even if he recovers from this acute illness. So, you might be asking why we have been and continue to be so aggressive in his care. Believe me I ask myself the same question dozens of times a day. But I've found that making the "right" decision isn't nearly as easy or obvious as when one is discussing a case study in the classroom or when I watched other families during my days as an ICU nurse. It's very challenging when multiple family members need to reach an agreement. Were it up to me alone we might have stopped all of this by now. But it's not just up to me. I certainly have felt and continue to feel quite conflicted because although he is deathly ill, he came into this an extremely healthy, strong, active man with good self-care habits. Although he has no living will (argh!!!), he did sign a consent for Peramavir treatment, an experimental influenza medication. This told us that he was willing to try edgy things and wanted a chance to get better. And probably the biggest consideration of all; that he is not some hypothetical patient—he is our big brother. And death is final. We don't want to lose him if there is a way to save him. We also feel sure that he did not realize just how very ill he was, until it was too late. After all, it was "just the flu." I will never take the flu for granted again.

I still have no idea how this will all end although my gut tells me he will not survive, but I want to be wrong. We are so grateful for the loving support and prayers of family and friends. I'm sure it's the only reason we are surviving this as well as we are. It's that "Footprints in the Sand" poem for sure. When the going gets too hard and we don't know how we can possibly continue, God holds us in his arms and carries us. I think we are being carried just now. It would just be too difficult to bear otherwise.

Rob really has an amazing team making an amazing effort. I notice that I keep using the word "amazing" but it's true. So many of the things I've seen and try to describe while troubling, distressing, and heartbreaking are also amazing. How Rob keeps hanging on in spite of so many significant complications and setbacks. How the doctors, nurses, and other members of the team keep working so very hard trying everything they can think of to help him. And how God gives us the strength to somehow endure and do what we must as we try to find our way down this road.

NOVEMBER 23, 2009

Rob coded this morning. His heart stopped and BP went to zero for about four minutes. Several members of the team were there at the time and were unable to identify any particular thing that triggered it. In any case they acted right away and restored his heart rate and BP quickly. This event earned him more vasoactive IV drips. Since then they've struggled to maintain his oxygen saturation level. The ECMO isn't working as well as before. The nurse said they will try "adjusting the ECMO" some more but she sounded discouraged compared with last night.

This is a journey we don't want to be on. I keep wanting to scream to the driver to stop the bus and let me off. I want to take Rob and everyone else with me. I don't like where this is going. But for reasons beyond our comprehension here we are. So, we keep doing what we we've done all along. We keep Rob and Mom in our prayers and support them as best we know how.

We try to hold on to hope that Rob might find a way to stay with us. But we also try to emotionally prepare (is there a way to do that?) for the very real possibility that he may not survive. So we are left trying to balance hope and some semblance of optimism with realism.

NOVEMBER 25, 2009

Last night we let Rob go. He fought so hard and so did his medical team. But it was too much for his body. In the end he had a huge stroke which was deemed unsurvivable and we knew that Rob would say, "Enough guys. I love you but it's time for me to go." I can't help but wonder if he'd spent the last ten days in conversation with Dale (my stepdad who died many years ago) and others deciding whether to go with them or stay with us. Ultimately he decided to go. God always answers prayer—but not always in the way we want or expect. Rob's was a spiritual healing.

All told, it's been a surreal two weeks of stress, worry, heartache, and difficult decisions. But also a time of coming together, of closeness, support, loving and being loved and being reminded of what is most important. Of the many gifts that Rob has given to us all I think that was one of the most important. A reminder that we are here to love and to learn. Relationships matter more than things. As we went through Rob's belongings this came home to me over and over. He left all of his things behind. He doesn't need them where he is. The only things I believe he was allowed to take with him were the lessons he's learned and the love in his heart for his family, his friends, and his God.

During the years I worked in ICU I saw families struggling every day with the same dilemma my family and I faced when Rob was ill. There were times I couldn't understand why they would let their loved one languish for so long on life support when it seemed crystal clear to my colleagues and me that death was a certainty. At times it even seemed selfish to see what they put their loved ones through. But when I walked that path myself I gained a much deeper understanding of what they were struggling with. It was a good reminder that it is so easy to oversimplify things when it is someone else's dilemma. But when it's ours (yours and mine) it is never as simple as others might think. Some decisions cannot be undone and when the responsibility for making that decision is on my shoulders or yours, the weight of the burden is astronomical. The very least the rest of us can do is remain patient and try to be sensitive to what the poor families are going through (and everyone, please write your living wills!).

Return to 2010

Amid the reality of my terminal diagnosis, I find that a recurring question that has arisen for me is whether a person can be realistic and also feel hopeful. Some seem to see the two as conflicting with one another. I have learned this is not the case, at least not for me. I've been able to acknowledge the reality of my diagnosis, to accept the fact that, medically and statistically, this will kill me sooner rather than later. Yet I've never felt so full of hope.

A Balancing Act

Many people I've talked with this last year seem to think that hope can only look one way. That I must believe I will be healed. If I fail to "claim" this healing they think my faith is weak. However, I've learned that hope can look many different ways. It might look like belief for physical healing. This occasionally happens. More often God heals spiritually. After all, how are any of us ever to go "home" to Him if we don't make the transition called death? Too often we see death as some sort of failure. I suspect God sees it differently.

Please don't ever think that just because a form of treatment "failed" that the patient or God "failed." Perhaps He was performing greater miracles in the process but we were just too fixated on physical healing and missed seeing them.

In the last year God has blessed me with so many forms of healing and small "miracles" for which I'm so grateful. There has been reconciliation in relationships, adjustment in priorities, and so much learning and spiritual growth for me and for others. Are these not miracles? Are they not reasons for hope?

So the greater question that has emerged for me is this: What does hope look like when you've been given a terminal diagnosis? I'm figuring the answer out for myself as each person must. For now, my cancer, though not gone, is in a holding pattern. So God is answering my prayer for "more time." That in itself is a miracle. And I am grateful.

∽

A friend and colleague from work told me that what she misses most in my absence is the "voice of reason" I contributed to our frequent faculty meetings. She said she always counted on me to speak up when nobody else would. When discussions seem to be leading us toward something I thought to be unwise I felt compelled to voice my concern. Furthermore, if I believed upper management was unsupportive or disrespectful toward us, I couldn't seem to stay silent. It's not that I wanted to be the vocal one or play "devil's advocate" but I knew that (probably) no one else would speak up on the issue and someone needed to. So it was often me. As a result, at work, I earned a reputation (at least in the minds of some) for being the realistic voice of common sense. Among those who disagreed with me I may have been known as the obnoxious one. At home among my family I became known for being opinionated. In all cases I was willing to take the risk rather than to remain silent.

My tendency toward pragmatism had a potent impact when I found myself diagnosed with stage IV cancer. What developed was an interesting inner dialogue in which I argued the merits of maintaining a realistic view versus that of grasping for what felt like false hope. It has been frustrating at times and enlightening at others. It would sometimes seem that if a patient reaches the final stage of acceptance, according to Elizabeth Kubler-Ross, they are viewed as depressed or having given up.[2] Yet, isn't the achievement of this final stage supposed to be a good thing?

Chapter 6: Notes

1. Viktor E. Frankl. *Man's Search for Meaning*. Beacon Press, Boston, 2006. p. 134.

2. Elizabeth Kübler-Ross. *On Death and Dying: What the Dying Have to Teach Doctors, Nurses, Clergy, and Their Own Families.* Scribner, New York, 1969. p. 112–137.

Chapter 7:
Trust

*Trust in the Lord with all your heart and lean not on your
own understanding; in all your ways submit to Him, and
He will make your paths straight.[1]*

What is trust? According to Merriam Webster it is belief in the
"assured reliance on the character, ability, strength, or truth of
someone or something." It includes having the ability to place confidence, hope, and even faith in that person or thing.[2]

Trusting in people is one thing. Trusting in God is quite another.
People have flaws and are known to disappoint. God is believed to
be infallible and is expected to never fail.

To tell the story about my current journey of trust in God, I must
go back in time to January 1999. I had just put my twenty-year-old son,
Brad, on an international flight to Townsville, a small city located on
the tropical coastline of Queensland, Australia. Walking back to the
car I found myself in tears. My younger son Brian, put his arm around
me and tried to reassure me that Brad would return in just six months.
But that was the problem. Somehow I knew that he wouldn't be coming
back. I'm not sure how I knew. Mother's intuition perhaps. But I knew
he was going for good and the thought was breaking my heart.

Brad had always been a young man of faith. Involvement in church activities, especially youth ministries was important to him. He had also been attending college and was a successful student, but lacked a clear focus. So when the opportunity to attend a six-month Discipleship Training School (DTS) program arose, he jumped at it. The DTS was sponsored by Youth With a Mission (YWAM), an international Christian missionary organization with bases all over the world. He knew it would buy him some time to figure out the direction of his life and also provide guidance as he clarified and strengthened his relationship with God and identified his life's purpose. I was proud of him but felt conflicted about his plans. I respected the strength and independence he was showing while having the same concerns any parent might. In the end, I realized that choosing to spend one's life serving God is such a noble goal that there was no way I could criticize or compete without sounding selfish and petty.

Brad loved YWAM and before long he also loved Melissa, a young woman on staff at the Townsville base. In their roles as student and staff member they were not allowed to pursue a romantic relationship. But as soon as the six month DTS ended, Brad decided to stay on indefinitely as a volunteer staff member and they began dating. Before long, they knew they were destined to spend the rest of their lives together. The very next Christmas, Brad brought Melissa home to meet our family and friends. It was easy for all of us to also fall in love with Melissa. She was (and is) an amazing young woman full of faith, integrity, and genuine kindness. I liked her right away and knew she would likely become my daughter-in-law. But I would be lying if I didn't confess to feeling conflicted about their relationship. It wasn't about Mel. I knew they would make a great team. It was the distance that bothered me. If we had been wealthy enough to fly across the Pacific any time we felt like it, I wouldn't have been so concerned. But I knew with my limited income and with their missionary income such visits would be few and far between. The distance was getting in the way of the life I'd envisioned where I would stay closely involved with my children and their children throughout the rest of my life.

The following Valentine's Day, Brad proposed to Melissa and they were married the next July. Their wedding provided my first opportunity to travel to Australia. My other children came too. I loved traveling with them and exploring the local area. I loved Townsville and its tropical location. I grew to love Melissa and her family. I loved that the staff members at the base provided a type of family support for Brad and Mel. I loved playing tourist on our three-day layover in Sydney. I loved everything about the entire trip, except for one thing: From where I lived, Townsville was ten thousand miles away which equaled approximately thirty hours travel time, four or five flights (depending on route), plus layovers and $1800-$2000 per ticket (minimum for coach at that time). This reinforced the fact that I couldn't just pop down for a long weekend. Trips there would require months, perhaps years of saving. And with their tight budget they could never afford trips home. This knowledge sent me spiraling into a state of grief for quite some time.

As the years went by I prayed, pondered, and cried over this issue. I knew I needed to simply accept how things were but couldn't seem to make myself do it. In a way that few understood, I was grieving the loss of my firstborn child. The day they called to share the great news that Melissa was pregnant, I cried for hours. But sadly, they were not entirely tears of joy. Don't get me wrong. I was excited and happy for them. I was excited to become a grandma. But I was also grieving the loss of the relationship I had envisioned I might have with my grandchild. I feared I would be nothing more to him than a photo on the refrigerator and I had wanted so much more.

Meanwhile Nicole and I had already planned a trip to Townsville in September 2004, before we knew of Mel's pregnancy. So when we arrived she was eight months along. I would have loved to stay for the delivery but my work commitments didn't allow for it. As it was we had a great time visiting with them. They gave us personally guided tours of the rain forest (amazing!), a crocodile farm (exciting and a little bit scary!), Paranella Park (so beautiful!), Magnetic Island (idyllic) with great snorkeling along the perimeter (fun!), and an afternoon looking for a duck-billed platypus (who refused to come out of hiding). The many perfect beaches put ours to shame (though I still love ours). There was soft, light sand, clear warm water and thousands of perfect tiny shells everywhere. It was magical. We had a terrific visit except for one thing. I noticed that every once in a while, a snippy comment would slip out of my mouth about how far away they lived, or how rare visits are, or the like. Each time I would see a look of pain on Melissa's face but she never made a comment. She was always polite, respectful, and gracious. By comparison I began to feel ashamed of my own behavior. I began to realize that I was putting a damper on the whole visit but couldn't seem to help it.

One day, when Brad and Melissa were attending a friend's wedding, Nicole and I decided to separate so we could each have a day to ourselves. I took a long walk to the Strand, a beautiful beachfront park that stretched for a good two miles along Townsville's tropical shoreline. The ocean view with Maggie (Magnetic Island) in the distance always captivated me. On that day I found myself crashing headfirst into my issues. I reached out to God as I was walking and crying and needing so desperately to resolve my feelings once and for all. Finally, I found myself sitting on the sandy beach just off the Strand, taking in the view. I tried to quiet myself so I might hear God's voice. In the process I found myself watching the seagulls, some on the beach and others in the air. There was nearly always a strong inland breeze and the seagulls loved riding it. One bird in particular was in a fairly relaxed state, wings spread, resting aloft on the wind. It appeared totally at peace. As I watched it, I heard God speak in his still small voice in the back of my mind, "See that? Now that's trust." As I continued watching the bird I realized it was putting complete trust in the wind; an invisible, yet powerful force that held it aloft without struggle, requiring very little effort on the bird's part. It just seemed to float in the air with a look of pure contentment. It wasn't trying to go anywhere. It simply soared in the air as the wind held it aloft in its magical way. Then I heard the voice again. This time He whispered "Trust Me." Two little words. I never expected the answer to my multitude of prayers to be so short and simple. When I was able to let it soak in, the impact was life-changing. For the first time in four and a half years I was able to fully relax and trust Brad to God's care. Since that day, the soaring seagull has become a powerful symbol for me.

So that was it. After struggling for so long and fearing I'd lost my son, here was my answer. It was simpler than I had expected, yet sweeter and more perfect. It was simply: "Trust Me." It wasn't the answer I wanted to hear. I wanted some booming voice that said something like "Your son will live in Australia a little longer and then move home to be near you where he belongs." But it was the answer I needed to hear. God knew that I needed to learn about trust. I didn't know what the future would bring, but He did. There were no promises that I would ever get what I wanted. No guarantees of anything. A simple request from God that I put my trust in Him.

For the remainder of our trip I was finally able to relax, enjoy the now, and not make any snide remarks about distance. After returning home I wrote a long letter to my son and his wife describing my struggle and how I had finally learned to hand them over to God and trust in His purpose. It was the beginning of a much healthier and closer relationship with both of them, in spite of the distance.

I cannot say it's all been easy since then, but God has brought that image to me again and again over the years and almost without failure when I've prayed for anything of significance His answer has been the same: "Trust Me."

A few years later, my brother Rob mailed me the aptly named book Jonathan Livingston Seagull. Sometime shortly after that, as I was boarding a plane, I looked up and oddly enough, there was a seagull sitting atop the plane just over the door. I swear he was looking at me as if to remind me about what it meant to trust in God. It felt like another confirmation.

So when Rob became gravely ill and died sometime later, you can imagine the answer that I heard to my many prayers. It wasn't the answer that I wanted to hear but it was the one that God knew I needed to hear. "Trust Me."

After my cancer diagnosis, when I began earnestly praying about my own health situation you can imagine the answer God provided . . . again . . . "Trust Me."

Over time God has built on this theme. First and foremost was always the foundational issue of Trust—but as other topics have been added they have created a powerful message.

Trust . . . Hope . . . Faith . . . Gratitude . . . Purpose . . . Reconciliation . . . Support . . . etc.

Trust relates to virtually every aspect of life; or can if we let it. I have always been grateful that God had led me to a profession that I loved, where I felt able to make a positive contribution. Although it's true that nobody goes into teaching to get rich, it offers many other rewards that make it so worthwhile. Unbeknownst to my students, over the years I kept nearly every single note, card, or letter of thanks. At work it was in my "special file" and now that I'm retired, I've added them to my personal "treasure box" at home. Anytime I feel down or wonder if my life has meant anything I can go through the many treasures I've collected and read my student's sweet words of appreciation. It serves as a reminder that I did sometimes make a difference, one student at a time.

Trusting God for Provision

Few areas of life require trust in God more than finances and provision. Ask most Americans what they worry about most and money will be at or near the top of the list. It seems there is always too little money and there are always too many bills. It's a rather sad commentary given the fact that the US is among the wealthiest countries on Earth. But there it is.

Finances have always been an area of struggle for me as well. So when I found myself needing to "retire" early by going on disability (something I never anticipated), I was naturally concerned about how I was going to continue paying my bills and especially how I would maintain healthcare coverage, which I needed now more than ever. So it all became an educational process for me as I learned how the COBRA act provides us with the right to maintain health insurance coverage for a given period of time after leaving a job. The catch was that I must make premium payments each month, which aren't cheap. But God came through for me. I had forgotten about a small insurance policy provided as an employee perk. When my friend in human resources reminded me of it and told me I could cash in half of it (due to health issues) it was just enough to pay the premiums through COBRA until I qualified for Medicare.

JOURNAL MARCH 2011
TRUST AND PROVISION

It's sometimes been scary not knowing if I will continue to have enough income to pay my bills and stay in my own home. But I keep telling myself that God knows my needs and He will provide. Funny how it all keeps bringing me back to the issue of trust. Imagine that. So I've been thinking about the word "provision" as God's way of taking care of us (provision = providing for). It made me curious to see what I might find in the Bible on the topic. I'm not exactly a daily Bible reader like some, but now and then I feel inspired to pick it up and read. I found several related verses but the one that most spoke to me was Matthew 6:33: "But seek first His kingdom and His righteousness, and all these things will be given to you as well.[3]

What I hear when I read this is that I don't need to worry so much about daily provision: food, shelter, clothing, money for bills, and so on. That if I keep my priorities straight and focus my energy on knowing and following God, He will come through for me by providing the things I need.

I've always hated completing forms and doing other paperwork. For some reason it feels challenging to me on a mental level, especially when they threaten to deny any requests if I make a single error. I heard from my employer's human resources department that I needed to get busy with the state disability application process. Although I supposed it will be a good thing to have it all done with, I found it overwhelming and confusing. I'd rather have a tooth pulled.

JOURNAL APRIL 2011
PROVISION

I know it will be a huge relief to have my Social Security Disability paperwork all sorted out and to one day be receiving disability checks but once again I feel overwhelmed with the application process. Even when I feel physically well I detest such things. I currently have so little energy; physical or emotional. I don't want to deal with it. But I know I must. I think I need help though. I need someone I know and trust to hold my hand and help me navigate this process. Someone who is smart, detail oriented, assertive, and patient (with me) and cares about my wellbeing . . . Oh what I wouldn't give to have Brad here for this. He is so good at this sort of thing. He would be the perfect man for the job. But alas. He is thousands of miles away. So whom else might I enlist? Please God send me the right person for this job.

It wasn't long before God answered my prayer, and as usual, it was in a manner I didn't expect. On Mother's day I received a surprising phone call from Brad telling me that he and Mel had felt God telling them that he should come spend some time with me. Their finances didn't permit the entire family to come but Brad had accrued enough air miles working with YWAM to buy a cheap ticket home. While here, he helped me complete the forms for state disability which helped me feel more confident that I was getting the information right. We had an awesome two weeks together and spent mother-son time like we hadn't had since he was a child. What a gift that was to me, on every level.

Shortly after Brad left I learned about a company that could help me with the Social Security application process. Not only did they take my case but they made a complex process quick and simple. As it turned out, my case was fast-tracked and I never went a single month without income. My total monthly income is not as much as what I earned at my job but it is sufficient for my needs. God asked me to trust Him and He provided just what I needed in a timely fashion. So I never went a month without health insurance or income. Talk about provision. I am so grateful.

I know my journey of learning to trust in God has just begun. I'm far from having it perfected. It's still easier to look back on past events and see how it all worked out than to maintain an equal level of trust regarding future events. I still find myself, at times, feeling anxious about my finances and less peaceful than I'd like about future health concerns. But this is when I remind myself that God has never let me down. He has me on this journey for a reason and I have a choice. I can give in to my anxiety and feel like a victim. I can feel helpless and sorry for myself and sink into a dark pit of worry. Or I can take a deep breath, blow off the anxiety and make a conscious choice to trust in God once again. He has been with me every step of the way. He will not abandon me now.

Chapter 7: Notes

1. Matthew 6:33, *The Holy Bible, New International Version.* Grand Rapids: Zondervan Publishing House, 1984.

2. Merriam-Webster: An Encyclopaedia Britannica Company, Accessed November 3, 2015, https://www.google.com/?gws_rd=ssl#q=trust+definition.

3. Proverbs 3:5-6, *The Holy Bible, New International Version.* Grand Rapids: Zondervan Publishing House, 1984.

Chapter 8:
Gratitude

"Piglet noticed that even though he had a Very Small Heart, it could hold a rather large amount of Gratitude." [1]

I recall countless occasions during my nursing career when I needed to help patients with very personal care, things like denture care, toileting, and bathing. It was usually a situation that made them feel uncomfortable. They felt vulnerable and embarrassed and hated being dependent on others for meeting their needs, especially with personal hygiene. Yet I noticed those who humbly accepted the care were the most contented patients. They often expressed deep gratitude for caregivers who were competent, caring, and willing to do whatever was needed. In comparison, those who resisted such care often masked their true feelings with anger and resentment. They were often the most unpleasant to be around, not only for nursing staff, but also for their own family and friends.

As for myself, I noticed at first that I was resistant to accepting help of any kind from others. It was a hard thing. It was humbling. I felt emotionally vulnerable. I felt I was imposing on others who already had enough to do. I didn't want to become a burden. I had been quite independent for so long that to give it up and accept help felt counterintuitive. But eventually it occurred to me that I could take the energy I was using to resist help and instead, learn to embrace it. Learning humility, I realized, might be a good thing.

I had several opportunities to practice this. Some were relatively easy, such as when someone dropped a meal by or ran an errand for me. But a greater personal challenge was the time I contracted a virus that caused severe diarrhea. This isn't a subject anyone wants to talk about, much less accept help with. But there I was running back and forth between bed and toilet, fully exhausted by the illness as well as the activity. My bedding needed changing because I hadn't moved fast enough on my last trip. I felt too embarrassed to ask anyone for help but realized I did not have the energy to do it myself. So I took a deep breath, reminded myself that learning humility was good for me, and called to my son and his wife in the other room.

"I really hate to ask this of you," I said rather sheepishly, "but I didn't get out of bed fast enough, and my sheets are soiled. Would you mind helping me change them?"

Their response was immediate and loving. "Sure, no problem at all," they said. "You just rest in your chair, and we will take care of it."

So I did. Emotionally, it was hard, yet as I forced myself to relax and accept their loving kindness, I felt the resistance melting away and deep gratitude taking its place.

Gratitude can be a magical and healing thing. I used to suspect this but now I know it for sure. Now I know why it was the second thing God said to me after "Trust Me." I've discovered that keeping gratitude in my heart makes it impossible for anger, resentment, or much sadness to take hold or reside there for long. Sometimes I forget. I become complacent and the negative thoughts and emotions creep in. It's easy to let that happen, especially when life is hard. But each time I remember to invite gratitude back into my heart, it chases the bad stuff away. It works every time.

Although I have written many journal entries about gratitude, there have been many additional times when I thanked God for gifts that I didn't write about. One of the great things about keeping a Gratitude Journal is that, like my treasure box of student notes and letters, I can flip it open any time I'm feeling down to remind myself of some of the many great things that have happened since I was diagnosed with cancer.

Focusing on gratitude has a magical way of dissolving depression, sadness, anger, or resentment. And writing about it is much more effective than simply making a list. Thinking (and writing) about each item takes more time and causes me to consider the when, where, who, and why of it. As I do so, my feelings of genuine gratitude increase.

Gratitude and Humility

I'm used to always being super busy. My daily mantra for years was "be productive." I couldn't stand to "waste time" or "do nothing." In fact, I became quite adept at multitasking so I could make the most of the too little time I always seemed to have. Now it seems that God is forcing me to do lots of "nothing." He's also teaching me to learn humility and accept the gifts that others want to provide.

A related lesson I've learned is that others often need to help. They are concerned and feel frustrated with their own inability to change the situation. They don't just want to help; they need to help, to do something that will make a positive impact. Therefore, I accept their generous offers not only for my own benefit, but for theirs as well.

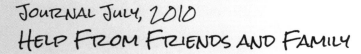

Journal July, 2010
Help From Friends and Family

On July 4, some work friends came over and totally renovated my front yard. And they came up with the idea on their own. It's now a joy to look out my windows and see my front yard. I enjoy the new landscape for sure. But more importantly, when I look at the changes, I am reminded of their thoughtfulness and willingness to spend their holiday helping me. Their actions were a perfect example of true thoughtfulness. They didn't just say, "Call us if you need anything." They didn't even ask if I needed anything. They simply said "We would like to do this for you on the fourth, if that's ok with you." It was totally ok with me and it was such a blessing to see them out digging in my flower beds, moving things around, and putting in new plants.

On July 5, family members came over. Some worked on my back yard while others cleaned inside the house. I wanted to join them but had no energy. I felt guilty doing nothing so I tried to help with a couple of small things and quickly exhausted myself. I had to spend most of the day on the sofa and even went to bed for an hour nap in the afternoon. It was weird and hard and humbling and wonderful.

As if this all weren't enough, now some of my nursing students from the college want to paint my house. I voiced some concerns to my supervisor. I didn't want to commit any ethical or legal violations. She reassured me that she had taken the issue "up the chain of command" and literally everyone supported the idea. To make sure, the faculty will pay for the paint and supplies.

Of course it would be awesome. My poor house has been

badly in need of a new paint job for several years. I even remember praying a couple of months ago that God would provide a way to get my exterior house renovated (yard, roof, gutters, paint job, etc.) in an economical way. Good grief! Have you heard the phrase, "Be careful what you ask for?" God is indeed answering my prayer but certainly not in the way I would have expected or even wanted. This past spring, I had professionals come and do the roof and gutters. Then I was diagnosed with cancer and was afraid to spend any more money. Yet God is faithful and has seen to it that my needs are being met. As is so often the case, He seems to enjoy surprising me by doing it in the least expected ways.

More Answered Prayer

God has answered many prayers through my sister who comes to visit as often as she can. She has the ability to connect with my kids in a way that few others can. They were all up late talking one night. I heard a fair bit of laughter from my room but I understand there were also lots tears. Stephenie reported that they had a "great conversation" in which each of my grown children voiced their feelings and concerns. They opened up with her in deeper ways than in the past and their shared thoughts creating a feeling of support and closeness among them. I felt so grateful to know they felt comfortable talking with her because they are often hesitant voicing their thoughts with me. Also noteworthy for me was to learn that their ability to cope well was closely tied to my own. One of them stated, "So far Mom is handling it well, so we are too," and the others agreed. I was glad to know this and felt motivated to continue coping as effectively as possible.

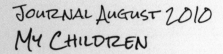

JOURNAL AUGUST 2010
MY CHILDREN

It is so awesome to have all three of my kids here together. It has happened so rarely over the past fifteen years. Brad and his family have come to visit for a few weeks. Brian and his wife are still four hours away, but they come for visits as their schedules allow. And my daughter lives nearby so from time to time I actually have all three of them here together.

I noticed years ago when I gave birth to each child it felt as though a piece of my heart and soul went with each of them. I can't explain it. I think it is just a part of the miracle of procreation and birth and motherhood. Since that happened I never felt totally, completely whole when they were away. I'm not complaining, mind you. It simply feels like a fact of my physical and spiritual biology. Anyway, each time that they've come together, over the years, I've felt a sense of wholeness and contentment that I only feel under these circumstances. It's not easy to describe. At any rate it is wonderful to feel this now, even if it is for a short time.

I'm not sure they see it but I believe there is a connection between the three of them that is nurtured when they are together. As their mom I so hope and pray they will continue to nurture that connection. I know they lead very different lives and I'm ok with that. But I also hope they come to appreciate what they have in each other. It happened with my own siblings as we grew older and it's something I treasure. I wish for the same for my grown children.

Solitude

My third and last child, Nicole, graduated from nursing school in 2006. She subsequently moved out to live on her own which left me with an empty nest. It was my first real experience living alone, and it wasn't easy at first. I didn't sleep well. The house was too quiet. I never felt like cooking for one. The feeling that something was missing left me feeling restless and unsettled. Somehow it even felt wrong to laugh at something funny on TV when it was just me sitting there alone; as if I needed someone else to confirm that it was indeed funny and justified my laughter.

Living alone definitely took some getting used to, but over time I did. I quickly tired of eating out and learned to cook for one. I'd make something I liked enough to eat more than once or I would freeze the rest. Either way it worked out so I only needed to cook about three times a week.

I learned many lessons as I lived alone, but probably the best one was that I learned that I am enough. I learned to enjoy my own company and I came to enjoy my solitude. I even learned the up side of traveling alone. I could go where I wanted when I wanted. I could eat what, where and when I liked, stay up late or go to bed early. I was in charge of my own money and could save or spend it as I deemed appropriate. No negotiations were needed. Of course there was also no one else to blame if I messed up, but I became okay with that too.

Of course there was a down side. Sometimes I wished I had someone to enjoy things with. But I didn't and I decided not to let that stop me. I occasionally felt alone but I rarely felt lonely. I'm sure it helped that my work kept me extremely busy and teaching assured that my work life was full of people. By the end of each day and by the weekend, I was ready for solitude. I found it restful and came to realize I enjoyed it as well.

After I was diagnosed with cancer, things reversed. Physical limitations forced me to quit work and I immediately became a homebody. In past years this would have bothered me and I'd have felt like climbing the walls after two days at home alone. But somehow under these new circumstances it was okay. I didn't have the energy I once did, so staying home and doing lots of "nothing" was just what I wanted. It's amazing how much my life changed. It might have been more difficult, but God saw it coming and knew I needed that time of learning to like my own company and learning to enjoy solitude.

Next came a time of allowing more people back into my personal space. Family from out of town came to visit more often and sometimes stayed for extended periods of time. I enjoyed this tremendously yet noticed that I still felt the need to retreat to my own space every so often to rest physically and mentally.

Then my middle son Brian and his wife, Sayo (SI-yo), moved to town and into the lower half of my house. We shared the kitchen but they really did most of the cooking. This was a good thing and ensured that I ate more than Ensure and cold cereal. They were also a huge help with laundry and other household chores. It was quite a change for me, but I was able to adjust and thanks to my lessons in gratitude and humility, was able to let them do these things for me.

One of the greatest blessings has been that each of my adult children, in their own way, has returned home to be closer, at least for a time. Brad and his family came from Australia for about five weeks during summer 2010, which was their longest visit to date. The goodbyes were painful, but having them here for that extended time was so worth it. Spending everyday time with each of them was a gift to my heart and had a healing effect for my body, mind, and spirit. Extended time to enjoy my role as grandma was a delight.

I recall one morning when all three of my Aussie grandsons, awake before their parents, came up to the kitchen on a breakfast mission. The only cereal they would consider eating was Fruity Pebbles and there was just barely enough left for the three of them. So I helped them all get set up with their bowls of cereal and toast after which they scampered happily back downstairs for cartoons. It was such a simple thing that many take for granted. But for me, someone who rarely (if ever) saw my grandkids, it was a moment I will always treasure. It was also a great reminder to me of what's most important. So often it's these everyday "little" things we mindlessly rush through that later become our remembered treasures. Then we wonder why we didn't recognize it at the time for the gem that it was so we might have soaked it up and appreciated it even more. It is the price we pay for our hectic lifestyles.

It is sadly common for Americans to get caught up in the rush and pressures of everyday life. We move so fast it sometimes feels as if everything is a blur. We make some things of greater importance in our lives than they deserve. Schedules, budgets, promotions, politics, recognition, prestige, reputations. In the mean time we lose track of some of the most valuable things: emotional intimacy, respect, appreciation, time for children, and expressions of love and support.

Of all the things we dread, I think it odd how we humans think the worst possible thing that could happen is to die. I've thought the same at times. But now I'm realizing this isn't so. I now know the worst that could happen would be to live a wasted life. A life of selfishness, focused on material "stuff," always thinking of myself. A life of wasted opportunities where I am presented with many open doors of possibility and I choose to ignore them all. God knows I've done this too much as it is. But now I feel more awake and hope to make better choices with my very limited time and energy.

My hope now is that I will find my way in achieving God's purpose for me during whatever time I have left. I believe what matters most in this life is whether we have learned and whether we have loved. I think that's God's purpose for us here—stated simply. So why do we complicate life and confuse ourselves by focusing on inconsequential things?

I've been thinking more lately about this gift of inoperable cancer God has given me. Some might see it as a curse—and I will admit there are moments when I feel overwhelmed, helpless, and sad. But most of the time I feel grateful. And I'm so grateful to feel grateful. Does that sound nuts? Even so, I'm still grateful. I could feel so much worse, if I allowed myself. And I know that people often do. I'm not saying that I'm better or smarter than any of them. I do understand those feelings. That's why I'm so grateful that God has shown me a path around them. It's called gratitude.

Have you ever noticed that it is difficult to feel sad, hopeless, angry, or resentful when you are busy feeling grateful? It's true. God has blessed me from the onset with a message about having an attitude of gratitude and while I haven't done it one hundred percent of the time, I think I've succeeded much of the time—and it really does make a difference. Whenever I notice myself feeling blue, all I need to do is thank God for some of the things I'm truly grateful for and the blues melt away. It's almost magical, but it's so real. There have been so many things that I'm grateful for that I could fill several books. So I will choose some of my favorites to share here with you.

Gratitude for Students and Friends!

My house is painted! What a strangely sweet, humbling experience. A small group of nursing students spent many hours prepping and painting my house over two weekends with paint paid for by faculty. These students who could have been home studying for their next exam or spending time with their own families wanted to do this for me. Larry, the project leader, used to do professional house painting, and he was amazing. I am so impressed by his work ethic and attention to detail. We nearly had to knock him off the ladder to make him take a break and eat lunch. He worked so hard and put so many hours into the project. A number of other students did too. Daniel came and spent several hours helping Larry pressure wash the house and then was also here all day Saturday along with his son. Many others were here all three days and some stayed until the very end helping Larry with all of the detail work and clean up. My Dean from work came by several times with supplies and food. It was an amazing group effort and now I have a beautiful, clean, almost-new-looking house. I feel so relieved and grateful to have it done.

I felt a bit guilty at times watching them work so hard on my behalf. I wanted to help them, and did a tiny bit, but I needed to carefully pace myself. I knew I needed to let them do this for me and for themselves. It was a tangible thing they could do to help me and I think it helped them too. Yet what an odd experience; to be on the receiving end of so much generosity, forcing myself to just relax and accept it, this is something new for me. I think it was part of God's plan somehow. Giving always feels easier than receiving. I've never had anyone do anything so huge for me before. It is certainly something I would never have asked of them; yet it was the perfect choice. I don't know what else they could have done that would have touched me or blessed me more.

Next my friends, students, colleagues, and even an administrator or two held a huge yard sale at the college to raise funds for me and another faculty member also facing a health crisis. I had no idea they were going to do this until the day before. It was an amazing gift of their time and energy. I've done yard sales before and know how much work they are. In addition, my dean happens to be a quilter, so she made a small, beautiful quilt and invited everyone to sign it which makes it feel so personal.

I feel so grateful and humble all at the same time. I've never experienced so much generosity. I don't feel worthy, but I surely do feel grateful.

JOURNAL AUGUST 2010
A NEW BED

After much thought I decided to spend my yard sale funds on a new bed. As time passed I began spending more time in or on my old bed and it was becoming more difficult to get or remain comfortable. I wanted to buy a twin-size, memory foam bed. However, they are quite expensive and given the changes in my finances, I was having difficulty justifying the expenditure. But thanks to everyone's amazing generosity, I was able to get the bed I really wanted, relatively guilt-free. It is making a huge difference and I am so grateful. My back and bum are grateful too.

I've enjoyed spending time with my daughter, Nicole, on her days off. She has done scrapbooking over the past couple of years so I asked her to help me on a project. I wanted to create a type of "gratitude book" that I could look through in the future when things get rough. She was quite agreeable to the idea. As I was clarifying my vision for the book I realized that most of what I feel grateful for are people, rather than things. Therefore, it has become a photo album.

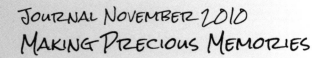

JOURNAL NOVEMBER 2010
MAKING PRECIOUS MEMORIES

Nicole and I spent the last thirty hours together working on our new project. We worked much of yesterday on my photo album, went to a doctor appointment, then to dinner at a favorite restaurant, and then out to a movie. It was a very full day and I enjoyed it immensely. The movie was funny and it felt so good to laugh. The food was good and I'm grateful I had enough of an appetite to enjoy it. Most precious of all was just the time with my daughter. I love her so very, very much. Words are not adequate. I found myself wanting to stop the clock when we were together because I know that these moments, as precious and sweet as they are, will turn into memories that will become bittersweet for her later. But what can we do? We both know that we are powerless to stop the clock. Our hearts ache at the thought of the separation that is inevitably going to come . . . . My heart breaks for her for what she will endure on my behalf. Yet I hope she knows what an amazing gift she is to me. Priceless, beyond description. I am so grateful to have her in my life.

Family visits have always been something I enjoyed. But now our time together feels even more precious. My siblings all lead remarkably busy lives, so getting time away to come visit me is not easy for them. Yet I see them each making an extra effort now. We've all stopped assuming that there will always be more time.

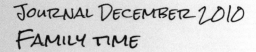

Journal December 2010
Family Time

I enjoyed a visit from my sister and her family who came from the Midwest to spend Thanksgiving with us. My brother-in-law was able to come along this time and I was so glad to have the opportunity to have a conversation with him similar to others I've had lately. I wanted to make sure he knows what he means to me and the impact he's had on our family. He is such a good man and, over the years, has truly become one of my brothers. He has a kind, gentle, caring nature, and his presence is always a comfort. He's one of those guys who doesn't say much but observes everything and quietly goes about taking care of things without needing to be asked.

I also enjoyed a visit with my brother Rick last night. He lives locally but is busier than most, so finding the time to be together is not an easy thing. I know he still hurts from losing our big brother. They were close playmates during the years we all grew up and he always looked up to him. And now he may be struggling the most of all my siblings to accept the gravity of my condition. But he is slowly processing it in his own way. Rick likes to tease and joke around a lot but in some ways he may be the most sensitive sibling I have. He's gone out of his way on many occasions to let me know that he loves me and is proud of my accomplishments. And though we've clashed many times in the past on social and political issues, we know that the love and concern we have for one another is strong. No matter what happens I know that I can always count on him to be there for me. Living nearby as he does, he seldom has occasion to write me. So when I received this sweet note in response to some good news about my medical tests, I knew it was a keeper.

"It is great to see more good news than bad. I know as mom says 'prayerfully-

carefully', we go forward, trusting that God will bring the answers to the prayers that weigh heavy on each one of our hearts. Sis, I know that within this last year the love that was always there within our family has deepened and grown stronger. There is nothing that can separate us from that love; and as Rob has, in my mind, so clearly shown us, love can reach us from beyond the doorway of death to let us know that it is eternally there for us. No matter where we are that love is always with us. I love you Sis, and I always will."

Christmas Letter

I sent out a Christmas letter in which I shared the loss of my brother and my cancer diagnosis. I then changed the tone of what began as a very somber letter by sharing some of the highlights of my journey which included profound lessons in trust and gratitude along with a few examples of some things I am grateful for. As soon as I sent it, I found myself wondering if I should have. Not that I really doubted the decision. It was more like that vulnerable feeling one has after baring one's soul. I keep wondering what God's purpose is for me now and I suspect this is a large piece of it: to bare my soul as I walk this path. Not that I'm an expert by any stretch at how to do this. But if others can see that I am somehow finding my way with God's help, then maybe they will feel a little less frightened and a bit more confident when their time comes.

My decision to send the letter was confirmed as a good one when the responses began rolling in. I received many heartfelt notes and letters of gratitude and have included below two of my favorites. The overall response helped me feel that I was on the right path, not only with how I'm learning to cope but also with my desire to someday share some of my journal writings with others.

"I wanted to thank you for the Christmas letter. I read and reread it several times. It expresses some things that I feel I have an understanding of but have a difficult time explaining in words.

I know everyone's experience is different, but I have felt the 'gift' of this disease in a similar way to what you described. It's very hard to express and I think people have a hard time understanding—no, I wouldn't wish cancer on anybody and I wish I didn't have to deal with it. Still, there is this side to the whole experience that makes life so sweet, so special. Focus changes to what really matters. The mundane little annoyances that plague our normal, everyday thoughts fade away as things like love, trust, family and gratefulness come into full view.

As I personally move on down the road of 'recovery' from cancer, I also feel this special awareness fading. I hope to hold onto the value God gave me through this, and your Christmas letter was a blessing that helped me revive this memory again. I am so glad you wrote it and I sincerely thank you."

~

"Sharon, thank you for writing your letter. How we face illness and our mortality says much about what we believe, in whom we believe, and what we learned on our journey. I am thankful and grateful that you know God's presence and can trust in Him. I know how difficult it is to figure out what to say in a letter to friends you rarely see when you write an annual letter: Do you write superficial things or get to the real heart of what your life and living is about? Having fought chronic illness and pain for twenty-seven years, I have had years I wrote and years I chose to be silent. I'm glad that you wrote. I'm sorry for your diagnosis and the loss of your brother.

I'm glad you have lived a rich life, with children, and that you know they are living their lives fully. Mostly, I am thankful that you have the eternal perspective and key to everlasting life. I know living each day through illness, doctor's offices, hospitals, tests, and diagnoses can be brutal. I personally look forward to heaven, where we get our new bodies and live without the scars of this earth. I have been reading a book called 90 Minutes in Heaven, where a pastor died, went to heaven, then was resuscitated; I also have a friend whose father died for a few minutes, then was resuscitated; he died about ten minutes later, after sharing what heaven was like those first few minutes. Her family was hugely blessed by the peace that came over him in those last minutes; he told them heaven was wonderful beyond our imagining and they should not worry for him. He was heading to a wonderful future. Few want to leave earth soon, and yet, I am eager for the joys of heaven."

~

As time passed and winter turned into spring, I continued to feel supported by family and friends. May brought the best Mother's Day celebration ever, which included strawberry waffles with my local kids and Mom and a phone call from Brad. I expected his call, but not his message. He was coming to visit in just ten days! What an awesome surprise! Thank you God!

May 2011

My time with Brad was a blessing. We didn't do much; just hung out together. We talked a lot, but also enjoyed sweet silence. We watched many episodes of NCIS (his favorite show) and I showed him how to play Candy Crush on his iPhone. As usual, saying good-bye was painful, and I now miss him deeply. But it wasn't as difficult as last time. I kept thinking of his wife and babies back home. His place is with them. Do I wish they lived closer? Of course. But it is what it is, and I am so grateful for the quality time we had together.

I also felt that the surprise of his visit, which I never expected, was a message from God to keep my attitude more positive. I can get discouraged and distracted looking at the many obstacles that keep us apart. But if God wills for us to be together, for whatever length of time, He will make it happen. So now instead of mourning his absence and worrying whether I will ever see him again, I keep my heart open to the possibilities.

It's been a full year since I was diagnosed with stage IV cancer. I remember wondering if I would live a year; if I would live to see the next Christmas, spring, and summer. The odds were not in my favor. But God is good. I think He's answering my prayers for more time, because I'm still here.

Every few months I undergo a chest CT and whole body bone scan. And thus far, each time I've heard the good news that nothing has changed. The cancer is not gone, but seems to be dormant (my word, not the doctor's). And each time afterward, I feel as though I can breathe better, emotionally speaking. I feel like I've been given permission to plan the next few months of my life. And each time I feel that my prayers for "more time" are being answered. He is doing it with modern medicine. Funny how some people think that things like faith, prayer, and healing are worlds apart from science and medicine. But I don't believe that. I think we often limit God by our own beliefs about what can and cannot happen. In any case I do not believe faith and trust in God need to be separate from faith in science and medicine. He is God of all. He can use science, medicine, and healthcare providers to do His work. I think He does so quite often. Sometimes He works with them. Sometimes He works in spite of them. Either way, God is God and He can answer prayer however He likes.

I am so grateful to still be here. To have the time with family that I love. And to have the opportunity to return to quilting.

JOURNAL AUGUST 2011
QUILTS AND BABIES

It feels so good to be quilting again, though my energy is low and progress is slow. I notice when I do it, how therapeutic it feels

Nicole's baby will be my first US grandbaby and I'm excited to be involved in the process. A special treat was going with her on ultrasound day. A little girl! At one point she put her fist to her mouth and started sucking on it and my heart melted. But as much as I loved seeing the screen, the best part was seeing the expression on Nicole's face. A combination of surprise, wonder, love, and excitement. One of my prayers had been that God would let me live long enough to see her become a mother. I saw the face of a mother that day.

Spending this special time with Nicole as she progresses through her pregnancy reminds me yet again that life is all about the journey and the lessons we learn along the way. So I'm trying to keep my heart open for what God would teach me so that I can make this last part of my journey as rich and full as possible.

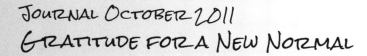

Journal October 2011
Gratitude for a New Normal

I've noticed that I journal less often these days which I think is probably a good thing. In looking back, I see that I wrote extensively in the beginning; nearly every day, then less frequently as time went by. Writing is a coping mechanism for me to deal with the stress (distress?) of my new diagnosis, so I think this indicates I'm feeling less distressed than before. I no longer wake up during the night worrying about how exactly I will die. I'm not always on the verge of tears as I seemed to be that first year. I feel more emotionally stable and, other than my complaints about chronic, severe fatigue, I feel content with my life. I actually feel as though I've achieved a new sense of "normal." It's not the same as the old "normal" and never will be, but I think it's a healthy "normal" all things considered.

Aside from a physician change, I have felt as though this "quiet time" (of non-journaling) indicated a time for me having learned to "just be." I spent time with family and a few friends, reading, and processing so many of the things I've learned since May 8, 2010. In fact, I didn't realize just how much I'd changed until I went back and read many of my early entries. I was clearly thrown off balance back then. I struggled with fears of death and dying, anticipatory grief at the thought of leaving my family, frustration at the response of some people to my diagnosis, and generally feeling overwhelmed. I felt as though I would never feel "normal" again. But the interesting thing is that I do feel normal again. It's a new normal for sure, but I feel as though I have regained my sense of balance.

Had I lived only a few weeks or months after my initial diagnosis I doubt that I would have had the chance to progress in this manner. I realize that many people don't have this time. I am grateful that God has granted it. It's helped me and I think it's helped my loved ones as well. It will still be hard for them when the time comes for me to leave but at least they have had the chance to watch me accept and come to terms with my new reality. I hope that knowing this, will ease some of their grief. Hopefully my acceptance has helped them begin to accept things as well.

Journal April 2012
Baby Girl!

I seldom journal lately but I have two great excuses. First, as already mentioned I'm on a steadier course emotionally and physically so that's all good. But the best reason of all is that I now spend most of my time, as energy allows, with Nicole and baby Reese. I was fortunate enough to be present when she was born in January, and have spent every moment possible with her and her mom since then.

Journal December 2012
Becoming a Grandma

I'd so looked forward to becoming a Grandma and developing relationships with each of my grandchildren. I had visions of spending time with each of them; baking cookies, doing craft projects, going on "dates" and such.

Funny how "life is what happens when we are busy making other plans." My first four grandchildren were born in Australia so for the past ten years there has been little contact. It's not accurate to say I didn't have a relationship with them. I did. But it was not the sort of relationship I had envisioned. It consisted of e-mails, poor quality Skype calls, exchange of a few letters and gifts and some real in-person visits that were awesome but few and far between and never long enough. I don't mean to whine, but I'm setting the stage for what I want to say next. It was what it was. It wasn't what I'd hoped for but I am grateful for what I got. In reality I felt as though I was mostly a grandma in name only. A photo on the refrigerator. A stranger they met every two or three years and then left before a real relationship had time to fully develop. But this past year I have been gifted with the opportunity to become a "real" grandma and it has been awesome.

An Extended Visit

Among the sweetest gifts I've ever received has been an extended visit from Brad and his family. They arrived the end of May 2012 and stayed until mid-January 2013. They lived in a house vacated by Brad's grandma who is now in an assisted living facility. This extended stay was enjoyed by the entire family and many friends. The older boys were able to experience riding on the big yellow bus to the same country school their dad attended as a child. We all celebrated each child's birthday as well as most of the major American holidays together. It was a light snow year but there was enough for them to make a snowman and do a bit of sledding. Since they lived only twenty-five minutes away there were many visits both ways and family gatherings. As I reflected on my time with them, I was reminded that relationships develop over time. Day to day activities and interaction are where relationships thrive and grow. Investments of time and energy, giving, sharing, helping, playing, being together, and so much more. My love for each family member grows as we spend time together. I love my grandsons for who they are. And I felt even more love (is that possible?) as I watched the loving relationships between them and their mum and their dad, my son. I recalled my mother once saying that she loved her grandchildren double, once for who they are, and again for being the child of her child. I understand that now.

JOURNAL JANUARY 2013
SAYING GOODBYE

It saddens me to know they will be leaving soon and to not know if or when I'll see them again. Now that we've developed real relationships I suspect I'll miss the boys even more than in the past. But it is worth whatever price I may pay. I'm so grateful for this gift of time and the chance to become a "real" grandma. I will think on this when I feel sad.

I hope they will all remember me later on, after I'm gone. But whether they do or they don't, I will know that we've had this time together; that it was real and meaningful and was a genuine part of their early childhood.

JOURNAL MAY 2013
REESE

Reese, Nicole's little girl, is sixteen months old today. Being with her makes my heart smile. I love watching her explore her world. She is so bright; she can watch me do something once and then she attempts to do it herself. Words are simply inadequate to describe the amazing little person she is and the joy she brings to my life. I often wonder whether she will remember me but try not to fixate on that. Right now she certainly knows who I am. When she sees me her eyes light up and she claps her hands. My heart melts once again and I soak up every moment with her I can get.

Roxy

This chapter would not be complete without a section about Roxy, my miniature schnauzer. I adopted her as a tiny puppy and she has kept me company for the past five years. She is quite a character, a great companion, and frequently makes me laugh. She reminds me of what a great example a dog is of what it means to live in the moment.

In the early months it was like having a new toddler in the house with potty training and all the rest. But as she matured we reached a point of great compatibility and it feels so right to have her here.

One of my favorite Roxy stories is about the day my friends at the college threw us a surprise party. I'd been invited to bring her to meet everyone at a regular Tuesday meeting. At the time she was still so small that she looked like a wind-up toy with great personality. She was quite shy for all of about ten seconds. Then she proceeded around the room getting acquainted with everyone. When it was time to open her gifts she was the hit of the party as she sniffed eagerly at each gift bag, then stepped inside and dragged each toy or goody out. She looked as if she'd been trained for this. Everyone was thoroughly charmed and we had a great time.

I later wrote them a letter of thanks for the many toys and treats they had blessed her with. One of her favorites was a little pink coat she wore non-stop for days after the party. Who knew she would be such a clothes diva? When I finally removed the coat for washing she gave me a funny look like, "What? You expect me to run around naked? I get cold!"

She loves going for walks or to the park. She also loves playing in "her" backyard (which is allowed) and barking at neighbors (which is not). She still loves chewing on things but fortunately has never chewed on furniture or shoes. She loves treats of all kinds and is especially fond of cheese and fruit, especially bananas.

Sometimes I worry how she will feel when I leave her. But it helps to remember that dogs live totally in the present and that Nicole and Reese will take good care of her when I'm gone. I believe that pets (when wanted and loved) can provide a powerful therapeutic benefit. Some pets are specially trained as "therapy pets" and are taken to hospitals, long-term-care centers, and other facilities just to spend time with patients. I'm so grateful to have my own "therapy" dog all to myself and I truly believe she is one of the reasons I've done as well as I have.

Notes: Chapter 8

1. A.A. Milne, Winnie-the-Pooh, https://www.goodreads.com/
    work/quotes/1225592-winnie-the-pooh (accessed 2/26/2017).

Chapter 9:
Changing Priorities

*When you die it does not mean that you lose to cancer.
You beat cancer by how you live, why you live, and the
manner in which you live.*[1]

One of the first changes I noticed in myself after my diagnosis was a subtle but significant shift in priorities. I suddenly found that material things had lost much of their appeal. As I looked around my house I noticed the stuff I'd spent years collecting didn't really matter anymore. I realized I didn't need most of the clothes in my closet so I had a clothing reduction day in which I sorted through my clothes and shoes and gave more than half away.

I'm not saying I never shop any more. Of course I do. I'm only human. But I do so less often and am more selective about what I buy. I just don't feel the compulsion to buy things to make myself happy anymore. I'm more likely to spend money on gifts for others or to buy simple things that enrich the quality or physical comfort of my life.

It's sad how much time and energy we Americans spend collecting stuff here in the US. We seem to have convinced ourselves it's the true course to real happiness. I fully admit there are a few things I really enjoy, like my recliner. It's the one chair in the house where I'm truly comfortable and it fits me. Having had triple digit temperatures this past summer, I admit that air conditioning is a nice luxury. A dependable car feels like a necessity, though less so since I resigned from work. There are so many things I could list: a comfortable house with doors that lock, a comfortable bed to sleep in, a sewing machine to mend and create things, a refrigerator to keep my food cold and safe, a stove to cook, a small freezer to safely store food, electricity and indoor plumbing. I could go on and on. Most of the things I mention aren't luxurious by American standards. But by most of the world's standards they are. In many parts of the world people don't have even a tiny percentage of what I have. I often remind myself that I've been blessed and am probably a little spoiled.

Stuff and Things

When talking with a friend one day about "stuff" she asked me to clarify what I meant. After answering her I pondered the issue more and decided to write about it here. These are my definitions and not likely what you will find in any dictionary.

Stuff and Things: two words which are sometimes used interchangeably. They refer to material things we humans feel compelled to accumulate; things we often value more than less tangible items that may be of much greater value. Stuff comes in many forms: cars, DVD players, clothes, toys, books, games, kitchen gadgets, etc. The list is endless. Many of us have a disturbing tendency to spend too much money on things we can't afford and often don't need. I suspect most of us lack insight into why we feel compelled to buy and accumulate all this stuff. It's often not for the actual utilitarian purpose of the item. Rather, many of us are somewhat addicted to the shopping experience itself. We use it as a form of entertainment and for some it may also be a dysfunctional form of therapy. A person is feeling bored, depressed, or restless. What to do? Go to the mall! Buy more things. And if it's a "bargain" then it's all the more attractive and the momentary pleasure from the shopping experience is even greater. In fact, I recall hearing that research studies had shown that the same part of the brain is stimulated by the shopping experience as is stimulated by drugs and alcohol in people with substance abuse disorders. It's a "fix" that feeds an unhealthy need. The problem is that the "high" obtained by shopping doesn't even last as long as the high from drugs. And it wasn't possession of the items that created the high. Rather it was the shopping experience itself. This explains why the novelty and excitement associated with the new item fades so quickly and why the person feels compelled to shop again so soon.

Many Americans seem to confuse the terms want and need. Furthermore, some fail to understand the value of delayed gratification. As a result, many conclude they need something simply because they want it. And they think they need it now. This sort of thinking is common among young children and I frequently see it in my young grandchildren. If they have the means and opportunity (and permission) they may impulsively buy said item right away. If not, they may obsess about it until they either get it, or become infatuated with a different item. Either way they often have an unrealistic idea that their lives will somehow feel more complete once they possess said item. This sort of thinking is normal among children. Responsible adults, usually the child's parents, endeavor to teach children the difference between want and need and also try to teach them the value of delayed gratification.

When my children were young, but old enough to begin handling money, one of the ways I determined how badly they wanted something was to ask if they were willing to pay for half of it themselves. If their answer was "yes" and if they were willing to work and save their money long enough to pay their share, then I knew their desire was sincere. Through this experience they learned that some things were worth working and waiting for (delayed gratification). Children who are immediately given whatever they want, whenever they want, may not learn this lesson and frequently go through life with an attitude of entitlement.

Adults who never learned these lessons may not have the insight to determine whether an item is truly needed or merely wanted. Furthermore, they become impulsive shoppers who purchase items, often on credit, that they cannot afford. Americans have become entirely too comfortable using credit cards. And often we delude ourselves into thinking that we can't pass up a bargain. What most fail to consider is that buying items on credit means that we end up paying a huge percentage in interest for however long the balance remains on our credit card. So much for the "bargain."

As the mountain of debt increases, we may become stressed or depressed. This may lead us to seek yet another "fix" to feel better, even if it's only temporary. I recall once buying (impulsively) and wearing (stupidly) a pin that said "I buy things I don't need with money I don't have to impress people I don't like." At the time I thought it was funny. Later I realized it was all too true and rather sad. I got rid of the pin. It took much longer to get rid of the debt.

I have another definition of stuff. This time it has to do with personal, emotional issues that we haven't dealt with. This is referred to by some as "emotional baggage." A pretty good name because we do in fact tote this baggage with us everywhere we go. It's impossible to put it down or separate ourselves from in it in any way until we've dealt with it. Dealing with my emotional stuff means that I am willing to honestly face it, try to understand where it came from and how it's affecting me and work through it in whatever ways I need to. If I do this effectively, and resolve the issue, then I can finally put it down. But if not, I continue toting it around for the rest of my life.

We have all kinds of emotional stuff. Much of it comes from the experiences of our early lives and influences us much more than we realize. Most of us are afraid to deal with it. Instead, we prefer to drag it along with us, every step of our lives, no matter how absurdly heavy it is, no matter how dysfunctional it is, no matter how it continues to undermine our efforts to be happy. We've somehow deluded ourselves into thinking that it is easier to drag this huge weight along and pretend it doesn't exist. It's sadly amazing how much energy we expend in this process. Imagine a one-hundred-pound woman dragging a two-hundred-pound suitcase of stuff that is chained to her. The key to the lock is in her pocket. She could use it at any time but is afraid to do so, because the key won't work unless she takes the time to deal with her issues. So instead, she drags it along, step by step, year after year. She pretends it's not there and expects others to do the same. If they mention it and suggest that she deal with it, her most likely response is denial or anger.

Some people are very good at dealing with their emotional stuff. Others, not so much. I've become better than I used to be, thank God. But I'd be lying if I said I was totally free of everything.

I believe (and apparently many professional therapists agree) that there is usually a connection between our emotional and physical stuff. A classic example is the hoarder. The person who feels compelled to literally fill their home with what most other people would call junk. To many of us, clearing it out seems like an obvious, simple solution. Yet it is anything but obvious or easy to the homeowner because their physical and emotional stuff are tied together. And unless they are willing to resolve the emotional stuff they may never permanently eliminate the physical stuff.

Journal August, 2010
Priority Shift

People die every day. Often they have no warning; no time to prepare; no last chance to say what's on their heart. Most of us go blindly through life pretending there will always be a tomorrow, thinking there will always be more time. All too often we put off saying and doing the things that really matter. In my case God has given me a wake-up call along with some time to do something about it. It has been such a gift to be able to spend quality time with family and friends. I have been able to create some sweet, tender moments with each of my children, my siblings, my mother, and other family and friends. These are my treasures now. The love I've given and received is so much more valuable than any of the things I could have accumulated. I believe that the love, the memories and the lessons are treasures I get to take with me when it's time. In comparison, I look around my house at the things I used to call my "treasures." Odd how they now hold so little attraction for me.

Why do we kid ourselves into thinking that if we can finally get the right house, car, clothes, or plasma TV, then we will finally be happy? Or if I just had the right body; if I could lose X number of pounds, or change my hair color, get a face lift, breast implants or any number of other things, then I will finally feel fulfilled. I will have arrived! We are such idiots sometimes. None of these things bring real, lasting fulfillment. I'm not saying that it's wrong to own things. But it is wrong to let our things own us.

Journal December 2010
Practical Issues

It's been great having sick leave to supplement my income but it will soon be gone. Shared sick leave helps but there's no guarantee about how long that will last. It really depends upon the kindness of others. That's a very humbling thing and makes me think of the many times when I could have made a contribution to others in some way and I chose not to. Yes, there were times when I did. But what stands out to me now are the times that I didn't. I feel like I've been so self-absorbed and self-centered my whole life. I always said to myself, someday when I'm not so busy I would like to do volunteer work and help others. Someday I will be able to give more, do more. Someday . . .

And even now, I still look at everything through the lens of my own situation, my illness, my pain, my fears, my issues. Even now I haven't changed so much and am embarrassed at what a selfish, self-centered person I am. I'd like to be more "other-focused" but not sure how to become so. Of course I've learned to do it in a very intentional way under specific circumstances. When teaching for example, or when providing nursing care to another person I'm pretty good at putting all of my personal issues on the back burner and really focusing on the person in front of me. But as a general rule, when I'm on my own time, I revert back to my "natural state" where I am the center of my own universe. This is not something I am proud of. It's just an observation.

Perhaps this is one of the ways where God makes a difference. If I keep Him as my center and focus more on Him then it forces a slight but significant shift where I move to the side just a little. This, then, impacts how I look at everything else. Slightly less from a "Me first" stance to a "What does God want of me in this situation?" stance. At least I hope so. It would be nice to understand this better and become better at doing it. It makes me think of the phrase "getting out of my own way."

A few years ago, I began carrying a water bottle with me every day to increase my water consumption. Now I hate to be without it. One day as I was drinking my clear, filtered, pure water I felt God speak to me about how blessed and fortunate I am to have such ready access to good water. He reminded me that millions on the planet are not so fortunate. That day I went online and found Water.org, an organization that works to help people build and maintain their own toilets and wells.[2] This allows them safe access to a sanitary place for elimination as well as safe, clean water for drinking, cleaning and cooking. I hadn't considered the impact such a thing could make. Because they now have safe water close at hand, they can use the time they used to spend procuring water to study or work. Because they no longer drink or use contaminated water, their incidence of water borne illness drops dramatically. This also increases their ability to work, study and be productive in other ways. Having a sanitary toilet close by reduces their risk of physical trauma from thieves, rapists or worse. Having a sanitary place for elimination significantly reduces their risk of communicable diseases. Being healthier reduces lost school and work time and increases their productivity. This all leads to increased physical and emotional health and well-being and ultimately helps them escape poverty. Lives are changed dramatically—from something as simple as clean water. I haven't looked at my water the same since. It's such a simple, basic thing and yet so very important.

Myth of the Bucket List

Funny how most people seem to think that if they are diagnosed with a terminal illness one of the first things they would do is create a bucket list of all the things they want to do before they die. Such lists typically include things like travel to exotic locations and jumping out of airplanes. What they fail to consider is that a person with a terminal illness often feels unwell and may have very little energy. This typically makes travel and high-energy activities unappealing. I noticed that when I feel this way, the place I most want to be is home, where I'm most comfortable, with my own bed, my little recliner, and my own bathroom. Furthermore, I also found that I most wanted to be with my family and very close friends. Why take off and leave the people I love when I most need them? Besides I can cover a lot of mileage on my laptop, sitting in my little recliner. It's cheap and I can nap when I want and don't have to share a bathroom. All in all, it's a pretty good deal. So a bucket list? Maybe for some, but I find that my real priorities keep me home close to family and friends.

Chapter 9: Notes

1. Nick Schwartz, http, "For the Win," USA Today Sports, January 4, 2015. //www.sheknows.com/entertainment/articles/1068465/ stuart-scott-10-inspirational-quotes-to-remember-the-espn-anchor.

2. water.org is an American nonprofit developmental aid organization resulting from the merger between H_2O Africa, co-founded by Matt Damon, and WaterPartners, co-founded by Gary White. Its goal is to provide aid to regions of developing countries that do not have access to safe drinking water and sanitation.

Chapter 10:
Purpose

The purpose of life is a life of purpose.[1]

Since being diagnosed with stage IV cancer I sometimes found myself wondering why. Not as in "Why me?" but just "Why?" as in, "Is there a special purpose in this?" I could have died any number of ways (and I guess I still could) but it seemed odd to me as a non-smoker and passionate tobacco opponent. There seems to be a bit too much irony in this for it to be a simple fluke. Additionally, there is the fact that I've continued to outlive my prognosis. I'm not complaining, mind you; I am very grateful. But I feel like there is a greater purpose in it than Him simply allowing me more time with loved ones.

Maybe it's just my egotistical nature and wanting to believe that somehow I am special. Maybe it's another version of the "Why me?" question; wanting to think I am too unique to die for no particular reason. Perhaps my asking God to show me the purpose was really me asking Him to create a purpose. If there is a deeper purpose, my desire to understand it would be consistent with my usual need to make the most of the crises in my life; to learn the most and grow as much as possible. I want the life I have left to be the richest, fullest experience possible and in the process, I want to make a maximum contribution.

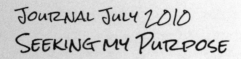

JOURNAL July 2010
SEEKING MY PURPOSE

It occurred to me today that my "purpose" in walking the cancer road may be to help my family (especially my kids) learn how to cope with pain, loss, and adversity. I realized that I can do this kicking, screaming, and whining (and I will probably do a bit of each) or I can do my best to trust God, focus on the positive, be grateful for what I have, and love others along the way. Either way it seems that I must go through this—so why not help my loved ones as much as possible in the process?

Courage

People often comment on how brave or courageous I am. It's an odd thing to me because I do not feel brave or courageous. Are they mistaken or am I? I'm simply trying to cope each day as positively as I can. I could bitch, and moan, and whine and the outcome would be the same. If I do, I'll make myself and everyone else more miserable in the process and that is surely something I don't want.

I wonder if anyone who is brave or courageous ever really feels that way. And what is courage really? I noticed two types of definitions of courage as I browsed through some dictionaries. One described people who are willing to take certain risks or perform dangerous activities without feeling fearful about it. This makes no sense to me. If they feel no fear, then how are they courageous?

Perhaps they are merely ignorant. Why would courage be needed in the absence of fear?

Another definition describes people who are afraid, who acknowledge the danger and have the option of avoiding the situation, but choose to act anyway. To me this is courageous. I may not feel courageous and am never sure how to respond when people say that I am. But maybe they see something positive (God willing) in me and they call it courage for lack of a better word.

Acceptance
January, 2011

About the time I think I've reached the "acceptance" stage I find myself again struggling to accept that what is, is. I have inoperable cancer. This is the reality of my situation. My prognosis is terminal. Fatal. Some days I struggle with this new reality and other days it feels surprisingly easy.

Suffering

Earlier today I spent time at the college in the nursing lab mentoring nursing students on suctioning, tracheostomy care, and other respiratory procedures. While there I found myself silently praying that I would not one day be their patient for the simple reason that I hope to never need a tracheostomy (artificial opening in the throat for breathing) or to be suctioned or to be on a ventilator. My living will should help to prevent this, but one cannot anticipate all eventualities and life is unpredictable. Sometimes I think, "Who am I to be hoping and praying to be spared from some of the very things my own patients have endured—things I have done to them?" Do I deserve to be spared from what they were not? Of course "deserving" may have nothing to do with it, but still, such thoughts go through my mind.

In some cases, the patients themselves or their family members asked that "everything" be done; and it was. Was it worth it? You'd have to ask them. Those who survived may well say "yes!" But others—those who died anyway—I'm not so sure. I cannot speak for them but I wondered then (and now) if they were praying in their minds and hearts that we would just let them go and end their suffering. I certainly wondered this with my brother. I felt so guilty about what we put him through. I understand my family's need to know that we did everything possible to save him but I felt so guilty that I was a part of doing to him what I knew I'd never want done to me. I just hoped and prayed that the drugs kept him comfortable so he didn't feel the awful things that were done in the effort to save him; things that no human should ever have to endure; things I surely don't want done to me.

A Purpose in Suffering

Although suffering is something that most people hope to avoid, myself included, there is some thought that voluntary suffering can serve a powerful, spiritual purpose. When I first heard of this notion I was doubtful. Yet the more I pondered it, the more it intrigued me. I couldn't understand how the suffering of an individual could translate into positive help for others, for society, or for the world. But then it occurred to me that this was exactly what occurred when Jesus voluntarily suffered and died on the cross. Most Christians know the story of the last days of Jesus when he underwent severe suffering of all types, physical, mental, emotional, and spiritual. He had the power and ability to avoid it, but willingly and voluntarily experienced it all for the benefit of his followers.

But when I consider regular people like patients I have known and certainly like myself, it seems more difficult to identify how it would work. Even so there are many accounts where "regular" people like you and I voluntarily suffered for the benefit of others. One of my (many) favorite authors, Dr. John Lerma, describes one of his hospice patients, a retired seventy-eight-year-old Catholic priest and university president with advanced cancer admitted to hospice care a short time before his death. He declined pain medication, stating that it was his desire to experience his pain in its most "raw" form. While at the university he had taught about suffering for spiritual freedom and believed that he now had the opportunity to live his beliefs through voluntary suffering as he approached death. He reported he was helped and supported in this process by angels who protected him and "sent love" to his heart. At some point in the process he reported that he no longer felt actual pain but instead felt enormous joy. He believed that on a physics level God had somehow transformed one to the other through an exchange of electrical ions.[2]

I do not claim to fully understand how this might work. I can only take his word for it. After all, he was the expert on his own body and he knew what he was feeling. It also occurred to me that the transformation of pain into joy may not be so very different from the transformation that I have experienced of fear, depression, and other negative emotions into the positive one of gratitude. It feels nearly magical, so I think it all may need to be a matter of faith.

I've come across this same notion, of voluntary suffering to help the world, in other places as well. Earlier in the same book, Dr. Lerma describes an amazing nine-year-old boy named Matthew who was blind and dying of a brain tumor. Frequently described as a child who was funny, loving, compassionate, and wise, he radiated love and joy to those around him. Mentally alert and lucid, he had refused all medications since admission.

He shared with the doctor that his angels had told him that if he chose not to be healed, his suffering and death would cause his mother's faith to be rekindled and that he could help his entire family and the world through his experiences. He also spoke about how angels helped with his pain and helped him escape his physical reality by taking him during his dreams to swim and play with dolphins.[3]

February, 2011
Grace Has Cancer Too

I recently learned that my very good friend from work has breast cancer. She will have surgery this week and then begin six weeks of radiation therapy. Fortunately, her prognosis is quite good. She confessed to feeling a bit conflicted about telling me this. I understand. I'd probably feel the same, were I in her shoes. But I am honestly relieved and happy for her. We are all terminal, after all, but I'm glad to know that her time here is not done. She has provided such great support for me. I'm happy to be able to return the favor.

Making a Contribution/Supporting Others

Walking this path better enables me to support others going through something similar. I believe I offer the therapeutic benefit of helping them to feel not alone. And while I'd prefer to not have experienced any of this, I do believe my experience enables me to provide better support than I would have otherwise. This somehow gives my own journey a bit more meaning.

Like many others I've always wanted to somehow "make a difference" in this world. I realize this is asking a great deal when one considers the size and population of the world. Perhaps making a difference to a few people in the world is more realistic. And perhaps that's enough.

Through much of my life I've tried to find ways to "make a difference" while also participating in activities that were personally interesting and rewarding. Thus my career in nursing and teaching although it's difficult to measure the impact one is having at the time. And now that I'm in a "forced" retirement and coming to grips with my own illness and mortality I've struggled to find new ways to continue this endeavor. For these reasons and more, as I found myself writing in my journal, at times I wondered if it was meant for another purpose aside from being an individual coping mechanism. I wondered if parts of it might be meant for other eyes, other people who struggle as I have, who might also feel frustrated with the lack of appropriate support groups, who browse bookshelves looking for someone, anyone, who seems to be on a similar path. Someone they can relate to so as to feel less lonely, less isolated.

With those thoughts in mind I began to pray about it and slowly I began to see in my mind's eye a book. A book that told my story yet was meant for others. A book that helped them to feel not alone, as I did upon finding the book by Walter Wingerin. A book filled with thoughts and ideas they might relate to. A book that might make them think "Yes! That's how I feel too." A book that included useful bits of information woven throughout. And most of all, a book that described, and maybe even inspired hope. But not necessarily the hope of survivorship. Those books already abound. Yet not everyone "survives" in the literal sense. This book would a different sort of hope. A hope for everyone, regardless of prognosis. For in the end, we all die. And most of us, at one point or another, are afraid. Most of us wonder about death; about what comes next.

And most of us wonder how we will make that transition, when the time comes.

Granted, this book doesn't answer all the questions one might have. But it does suggest a few answers. And, more important, it offers reasons for hope regardless of prognosis. And it might offer another reason for why I'm still here now, writing this down.

I also envision a day in the future when someone reads this book after I'm gone and as a result finds himself or herself feeling less alone and more hopeful.

Perhaps you are that person. And if you are, I am grateful.

Chapter 10 Notes

1. Gallup.com/poll/1654/honesty-ethics-professions.aspx, accessed 5/19/2017

2. John Lerma. *Into the Light: Real Life Stories About Angelic Visits, Visions of the Afterlife, and Other Pre-Death Experiences.* Kindle locations 1023-1028.

3. Ibid, Kindle location 150-174.

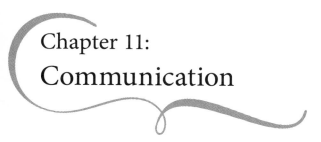

Chapter 11:
Communication

The single biggest problem in communication is the illusion that it has taken place.[1]

Issues of Trust

There are certain relationships in which a basic level of trust is granted right from the start. For example, when asked whom they trust above all, Americans in a 2016 Gallup poll revealed that they place nurses highest (for the eleventh year in a row), followed by pharmacists and the doctors.[2]

As a nurse I found this gratifying. Yet it also reminded me of the great responsibility all healthcare professionals bear, for this trust is sacred and must not be taken for granted or betrayed. The public, in general, is willing to extend us a large amount of trust simply based on the professional positions we have attained. When our behavior meets or exceeds expectations, trust is maintained and even increased. But if patients believe they have been disrespected, lied to, or betrayed in any manner, trust levels plummet, often beyond repair.

Truth Telling

Physicians need to be able to trust that their patients will honestly answer health-related questions including but not limited to their primary complaint, medical history, social history, and symptoms. Accurate information is particularly important for the physician to reach the most accurate diagnosis and plan appropriate medical care.

Patients also need to be able to trust that their doctors will be fully honest with them in every aspect of their care, including but not limited to diagnosis, prognosis, and test results. The only exception to this may be when patients or family members have stated they do not wish to be fully informed. This might occur because of religious beliefs, cultural customs, or personal preferences.

All physicians, especially oncologists, must choose their words carefully as they consider the patient's position of vulnerability in light of their own positions of power. Words spoken carelessly can dash patient's hopes. A key point to remember is how one defines hope. If physician and patient both believe hope only exists when a cure is possible, then no wonder they sometimes go to great lengths to avoid honest conversation and dance around the D words (death and dying). If both patient and doctor believe in the power and possibilities of hope, regardless of prognosis, then the door is wide open to conversations regarding what the patient is hoping for and how they can work together to achieve those goals. If only the patient believes in the power of hope, regardless of prognosis, then he or she can inform the doctor and set the direction for future conversations and goal setting. If only the doctor is the believer, then she or he must be sensitive and empathetic but can still inquire about what hopes the patient has. This may allow for some collaboration between patient, physician, and loved ones to enable the fulfillment of some of those hopes.

While honesty should be the general rule, brutal honesty is not necessary as it may cause the patient unnecessary emotional pain. Failure to tell a patient the complete truth may be considered lying by omission and the doctor may later find him or herself accused of withholding critical information or instilling false hope.

Historically, doctors and patients often participated in a charade where doctors told terminally ill patients incomplete truths. Patients were then expected to pretend their illness was not fatal and to do as they were told. Then patients underwent treatment after treatment until they reached a point where they could no longer deny the reality of their impending death. As they became weaker they became fully aware of the real truth while those around them continued on with the charade. This left patients feeling alone and isolated.

Fortunately, today most doctors tell patients when their cancer is not curable although they sometimes fail to state this clearly enough for patients to fully understand. Furthermore many are still hesitant to clearly discuss the actual prognosis, especially when it is poor. I understand this to a certain extent. It is a difficult subject to broach and doctors are not God (despite rumors to the contrary) and cannot know precisely when a patient will die. In any case they tend to fall into one of two categories. The first are doctors who are brutally honest to the point of being harsh and hurtful. An example might be the physician who tells his patient she has "only six months to live if she is lucky" so there is "no point in considering further treatment." The second, much larger category of doctors, are those reluctant to discuss prognosis and avoid mention of the D words whenever possible. Instead they tend to veer into their own comfort zone which involves discussion of available treatments, even when options are few and far between and unlikely to help.

Another consideration is that some patients do not want to know or do not like the idea of another person (even a doctor) putting an "expiration date" on their life. Because of all these factors, physicians have a tendency to over-estimate the length of time patients have to live. Is this wishful thinking? Is it a positive, glass half full perspective? Or is it just easier to discuss this dreaded topic if they embellish a bit and add some extra time? I'm thinking it's probably all three but I suspect it's mostly the last one. Even so, Gwande notes that when quantifying the amount of time that might be bought through treatment, physicians are generally thinking in terms of a year or two while patients are thinking more like ten or twenty years. That's quite a discrepancy in expectations. Now add to this the fact that "more than forty percent of oncologists admit to offering treatments they believe are unlikely to work" and the expectation gap widens further.[3] When I came across the above statistic my response was "Seriously? Forty percent! OMG!" It made me think back to my IV chemo experience that first summer of 2010 and I couldn't help but wonder what was in my doctor's mind at the time. Then we discovered my tumor had an antigen sensitive to targeted cell therapy and my doctor prescribed Tarceva. I actually remember him saying that he felt like, "for the first time really, [he had] something to offer that might help." So it made me wonder if he knew from the beginning that the other stuff wasn't likely to help. Was he part of that forty percent? Did he really think I would prefer to go through the hell of chemotherapy than do nothing? If it had a real chance of helping, I'd consider it. But if it didn't I'm not the sort that would do it just to be "doing something."

Before I go putting all the blame on my (or any) doctor, there is something else to be considered. We (patients and loved ones in general) heap a huge burden of expectation on our doctors. Rarely do we speak right up and tell them we don't want to take any treatments deemed unlikely to be effective. Most of us, when first diagnosed, are shell-shocked, overwhelmed, and frightened, and ask our doctors some variation of the following: "What can be done?" "Can you fix this?" "Can you help me?" "There must be something you can do." "I'm not ready to die." Now put yourself in the doctor's shoes. How do you suppose you would respond?

I think doctors avoid talking prognosis and prefer to discuss treatments, even ineffective ones, because it feels much easier than discussing a grim prognosis, especially if the doctor's only concept of hope means physical cure. Furthermore, that is what they believe we expect. Patients expect to be cured, or at the very least, given more time. Much more time. Rarely do patients want to discuss any other possibilities and they don't want a doctor whom they perceive has "given up" on them. So we must all take some responsibility for the communication gap, doctors, patients, and even loved ones.

Now having said that, I will say this. Doctors, being the professionals, need to put on their big boy (or big girl) pants and discuss prognosis if this is a conversation patients are willing to have. If or when they believe further (or any) treatment is futile physicians need to fess up and be honest. Some patients (and families) won't like it. But I think some will find it refreshing. Furthermore, they should be reminded that they are free to seek a second opinion. Integrity is everything and integrity requires honesty. I will concede that few patients are ready to absorb much information on that first visit. But what about the second, third, or fourth visit? Somewhere along the line, sooner rather than later, patients need to hear the truth.

Another reason physicians may be reluctant to talk prognosis is they may underestimate what their patients can emotionally handle. Yet they need to know that by trying to "spare" patients and let them "hang on to hope for a little while longer" they may unwittingly be robbing them of the opportunity to explore what real hope is for them. Reluctance to discuss the truth may also rob patients of precious time to take care of business and reconcile relationships. People are often capable of much more than they are given credit for. When doctors express confidence in their patients' personal faith, strength of character and coping ability, patients often rise to the occasion to do what they must. This is especially true when physicians inform them of the strong support network available to them in the form of hospice and palliative care (which will be discussed in chapter 12, Pain).

The Language of Warfare

Everyone talks about cancer as a *battle* that must be overcome, and about cancer patients whose treatments were ineffective as having failed. I've always been uncomfortable with using military language (in reference to cancer) and it took me a while to sort out my feelings on the matter. Among patients, medical people, and even the general population, we frequently hear statements like:

The patient failed to respond . . .
She lost her battle with cancer . . .
You must fight this!
You must not let it win!

I'm not sure I agree. For me cancer is not a battle, death is not a failure, and cancer patients don't fail, although the treatment may. Personally, I don't think we should use the word failure at all. It frames the entire process in a negative light when there are so many positive lessons to be had.

While shopping at a local bookstore this book caught my eye: Letters from the Land of Cancer by Walter Wangerin Jr.[4] I read a page or two and found myself in tears. I dried my eyes and tucked the book under my arm knowing I dare not open it again until I was home where I could (if need be) cry in private.

The author's rich history includes serving as an intercity pastor, a speaker for a radio program and authoring forty books. In spite of having lung cancer he is currently an active university research professor. The book I found seems to be one of his lesser known works but was the first thing I'd found that spoke to my heart in a real way. The first words to catch my eyes were, "This kind of cancer doesn't go away. It will kill you." I suppose the words were quite blunt, but at that point I was thirsty for someone who would use blunt language. The author wasn't on the survivorship bandwagon preaching about the power of positive thinking. He was speaking the truth as he saw it. His truth.

Like myself Mr. Wangerin seems to feel conflicted when so many people encourage him to "fight" and use the military warfare paradigm. He actually had one older woman proclaim that his cancer came from the devil and that he should pray until the "evil spirits" left him.[5] Wow! I expect she thought she was being supportive. I suppose she was using the spiritual warfare paradigm which is also quite common. They are both epidemic.

JOURNAL JANUARY 2011
MORE WANGERIN

God Bless Walter Wangerin Jr., for in spite of his frustrations with what other people may say or do, he finds a way to extend them grace by stating "I put myself in the shoes of those who feel unable to put themselves into mine."[6] What a generous heart he has.

Wangerin too noticed the common obituary themes about people having experienced a "long battle with cancer" and he wondered as I have, why we feel compelled to cast patients as soldiers, knights, or warriors.[7] It makes them sound noble though I don't know why that would be necessary. More to the point, if they won the battle, they apparently fought well. But if they lost the battle (died), then what? Perhaps we need to redefine what it means to win and to lose, at least within the context of cancer. For sooner or later we all die.

When I've tried to voice my thoughts around this, others often misinterpret it as a sign that I've "given up" and have "decided to die." But that's not it. I simply believe there is another way, a different context in which to view this.

I view it all as a part of the person's life journey. When we use words like *battle*, *fight*, and *fail*, we cast a negative shadow over the entire journey. As our fears and anxieties infuse our language the illness becomes larger than life and we descend into despair. So, rather than focusing on the cancer, I believe we should look at the positive aspects of the *journey* and note the many **gifts, blessings**, and *miracles* along the way. Rather than emphasizing the disease, let's notice the person and his or her response. What lessons were learned? In what ways did she grow? How were his relationships impacted? Whether or not the patient dies, there are lessons and insights to be had and love to be expressed. Death is a natural part of life, a process that leads to something more. How can it be a failure when the last days are rich and filled with love, when the dying person gains new insights and experiences spiritual growth?

To some it may seem to be a matter of semantics but I think it's so much more. The language we use reflects our core beliefs. Our words become statements of our intent. And we proceed to manifest what we've stated.

Many of those who overcome their cancer in the short term, will experience its return or succumb to something else one day. For we are all human and this means that we are all terminal. If we view death as the ultimate failure, then we've predetermined that we all will fail. Why do we do this to ourselves?

Semantics

As I pondered this idea of using different language it occurred to me that words I'd like to use in place of battle or fight might be struggle or challenge, or better yet opportunity. Some laugh when I use this word. But in using it I remind myself that I am not a victim and I can choose my response. This is where I have the power to exert some control over the situation. I may not always be able to control life circumstances or what happens to me. But I always have the ability to determine my response. And if I seek positive responses things turn out far better than if I'd merely reacted without thinking.

If I remind myself that it's really an opportunity, then I'm more inclined to listen for that still, small voice that helps me see the silver linings around each cloud. And inevitably I hear it, I see it, and I learn. Gratitude follows and I'm okay once again.

I've noticed that it has always been during times of adversity that I've learned and grown the most. These times are where I find the pearls that life has to offer. But it usually takes conscious intent to find them. It rarely happens by accident. So it is in the act of remaining conscious, reflecting on my experiences, and doing the necessary work, where learning and growth occurs. And it does require work. Honestly looking at myself is not easy. I become acutely aware of the flaws, imperfections, and blemishes on my character. Acknowledging these parts of myself is more than uncomfortable. It's downright embarrassing, painful even. Yet it affords me the chance to work on removing and replacing them.

By flaws and blemishes I really mean ineffective and unpleasant habits, reactions and behaviors, ways of being and doing that do not earn the results I want. The thoughtless things I say and do that get me into trouble or at the very least, do not achieve the results I want. As I admit to such things I have the opportunity to replace them with more effective ones. And as I begin to tryout more effective ways of responding, I note which ones help me to achieve the more positive results I wish for. This process rarely comes naturally or easily, but the results are so worthwhile

Many years ago, I had the chance to attend a series of workshops.[8] A friend recommended them, saying they would afford me the chance to get to know myself better than ever and to be more successful in getting the results in life that I most wanted. So I signed up and went to the first one feeling excited and a little bit anxious. It turned out to be the best gift I have ever given myself. Throughout the three-part series there were many fun activities including large group discussion, small group activities, one-on-one conversations, role playing, games, short meditation-like sessions, and much more. I made many friends, identified my own personality/leadership style, and learned to recognize the personality/leadership style of others. This alone made a hugely positive impact on my understanding of and communication with others. I also set personal and professional goals, wrote my own definition of success, learned to become a better listener, learned more about providing true support within relationships, learned how to better give and accept sincere complements, and developed and replaced old ineffective coping skills with newer healthier ones. It was all a great deal of fun but was also a great deal of work. Noticing unattractive behaviors in myself is not pleasant. But replacing them with better ones and seeing new results is so rewarding.

A simple, but useful example is that I noticed my own annoying (to others) habit of talking on top of others (interrupting and speaking before they are done speaking). I still struggle with this, but am much more likely to notice when I'm doing it. Then I quickly apologize and remain quiet while they finish their thought. This sort of etiquette is much more conducive to healthy relationships and less likely to offend others.

Another example is changing from "you" language to "I" language in which I own my own actions, thoughts, and feelings. This manner of speech is so common that you probably don't notice it. But make a point to notice the next time you hear someone speaking about an exciting or distressing experience how often they say "you" when they really mean "me." I've become so aware of it that it now annoys me to hear others use it. However, I usually resist the temptation to say anything and simply focus on their message. The advantage to using "I" language is that it's a more powerful way to speak because it allows you to really own your ideas and feelings. I challenge you to try it. It may feel foreign and a bit awkward at first, but in time it becomes quite natural.

One last example is about noticing when I'm acting like a victim. The triggering situation might be as simple as another driver "stealing" the parking space I had my eye on. Or it might be as complex as learning my spouse has been unfaithful and the subsequent demise of my marriage. In either case I can take on the victim identity, feel angry at the other person and very sorry for myself. In general, it is a stance in which I believe that some other person, or group of people, or even God has knowingly attacked or hurt me in some manner. I may have a whole pile of reasons why I believe this is so and love to recite to others in order to convince them that someone or something else is guilty and I am innocent. Some or all of it may even be true. But the problem with this sort of thinking is that it absolves me of any responsibility for helping to create the situation in which I currently find myself. And if I believe I did nothing wrong then I don't need to change. I may be off the hook now but I've also robbed myself of the opportunity to learn and grow.

On the other hand, if I am honest I must admit that I didn't have any greater right to the parking space than anyone else. I also concede that we are all simply going about our day doing the best we can. The other driver most likely didn't think about me one way or another and was just grateful as I would have been to have found a space. His need may even have been greater than mine. Or maybe not. The point is that I don't know and it really doesn't matter. What would matter and be totally absurd would be for me to become angry and let it spoil my day. Or worse yet, become vindictive and try to get some form of revenge by vandalizing his car. I realize this sounds foolish and childish, but this and other forms of road rage are all too common.

The situation with an unfaithful spouse is much more complex and covers a much larger time frame. I will admit to feeling quite betrayed, hurt, and angry for a time. But I knew that in order to heal as quickly as possible, and get on with my life I needed to let go of my victim identity and admit to myself that there were ways in which I also contributed to the demise of my marriage. When I found myself consumed with anger or other negative feelings I left the house for a brisk walk or confided in a close friend. I found exercise to be especially therapeutic and spared my kids and friends from enduring even more of my rants than they already had. I also found journaling (like I do now) to be quite therapeutic and helpful in clarifying my thoughts. Other lessons learned were too numerous to describe but I recall repeating to myself many times that "I'm not gonna go through this hell for nothing! So I'm gonna milk this sucker for all it's worth (lesson-wise) and learn as much as I can." And I did. And eventually I came to believe that adversities and sometimes even tragedies become missed opportunities if I fail to learn and grow from them. And that's been my mantra every time I've met with adversity since that time.

Throughout life we are given an endless array of opportunities for learning and growth. Yet all too often we plod along in a semiconscious state, partially blind and unaware letting golden moments pass us by. Now more than ever, I want to remain awake and aware. I want to see, to notice and to learn. Yet my energy is low and often I simply coast along with my mind in neutral and my body at rest. I know this is okay at times and can be part of the self-care I need. But I don't want to miss the opportunities and lessons that God has ready for me. So this is the struggle. To remain awake and invest my energies into what matters most.

I think perhaps, that when people focus on the battle with cancer, they are externalizing the struggle and making cancer the enemy. I wonder if they feel this excuses them from any obligation or responsibility to do the inner work that is so much more important. In an odd way, it becomes its own form of denial.

Damaging Language

Language is one of our key forms of communication. With this in mind it's important to understand key terms often employed by physicians. Informed consent is a medical and legal term that refers to a healthcare provider's obligation to provide all relevant information to the patient who is choosing among treatment options. This includes potential risks and benefits of the treatment being considered and other treatment options available, including risks and benefits of each as well as risks and benefits of no treatment at all.

Patients who are deemed to be resistant to following medical advice or who fail to use medications as directed are sometimes labeled as recalcitrant (disobedient or unmanageable) or noncompliant (rebellious or uncooperative). Either term paints a negative, childish picture of a patient who simply won't do as he or she is told.[9] This is unfair to patients who always have a reason for their behavior but may be uneasy or too embarrassed to discuss it with the doctor or nurse. There are numerous reasons patients might not follow instructions. These include, but are not limited to, failure to understand, inability to read, unacceptable side effects, financial concerns, and cultural or religious beliefs. Rather than labeling patients as uncooperative it would be far better for physicians to make a sensitive attempt to understand their patients' concerns. There's a good chance the issue can be resolved while keeping the patient-physician relationship intact. With the same goal in mind, patients can help build this relationship by communicating clearly with their physician about their priorities, fears, and concerns.

Failure to Clarify

All health care providers must remember that few patients have studied anatomy or medical terminology and most do not understand the language. For this reason, physicians should take extra care to use common language when speaking to patients and always check for full understanding. Simply asking if they understand isn't an adequate way to evaluate understanding. It's better to ask the patient to paraphrase the information (state in his or her own words). This allows the doctor or nurse to verify or clarify as needed. Each medical specialty has a language of its own and oncology is no different. A few terms common to this area and of great importance to clear communication include the following:[10]

- cure: indicates the treatment, medication, or procedure will eliminate the disease and it will not return. An example is treating a common infection like strep throat with an antibiotic. If the patient completes a full course of an appropriate antibiotic as instructed, the infection should go away.

- palliation: the treatment, medication, or procedure will not provide a cure but is being done to help relieve pain or other symptoms and improve quality of life.

- partial remission: This term may be used when cancerous tumors and lesions have shrunk to fifty percent or less of their original size. It indicates improvement and progress and may be reason for hope. However, it does not mean cure or complete remission and the tumor could begin to grow again at any time.

- complete remission: Indicates the cancerous tumor and lesions are no longer detected by any tests. It does not mean cure but does indicate great progress and may certainly be reason to celebrate. However, return of certain types of cancer is common after a period of time. Therefore, a complete remission may be great progress on the road to a cure or may simply be an extension of the patient's life span before the cancer returns. Subsequent remissions after the first one may or may not occur.

Failure of the physician to clarify the difference between cure and remission or between a full and partial remission can result in a huge misunderstanding. Once patients discovers the discrepancy they will be more upset than if they'd been told the truth from the beginning. They may believe the physician intentionally failed to clarify, which for some is the same as a lie. Even if the physician spoke with good intentions, trust may be gone and the patient may feel betrayed and unlikely to ever believe the physician again. Groopman states that any evasions in an effort to promote hope may be tempting but only serve to fulfill an illusion which provides only hollow hope.[11]

During his residency, Dr. Groopman supplemented his income by moonlighting at a small practice where he covered the patients of a Dr. Keyes during his time off. He was in the office one day with Dr. Keyes when he met fifty-three-year-old Francis who had been diagnosed with advanced colon cancer. As he observed Dr. Keyes's interaction with the patient, Groopman noticed that he never explained that the cancer would kill her. Further, he never used words like fatal or terminal and emphasized only positive information stating, "All of the cancer was removed from your bowel and the surrounding lymph nodes. A few small spots of tumor were found on the left side of the liver. But we have chemotherapy to help take care of them . . . The chemotherapy continues until we shrink the remaining cancer down." By her expression of obvious relief Groopman concluded that the patient believed she would be cured. He also knew the patient might or might not benefit (live longer) from the chemotherapy, but this was never explained to her. After the patient left, Dr. Keyes explained that he believed it was best to not give more information since it would "overwhelm her" and "make her remaining time even more miserable." Three months later as Dr. Keyes showed her the new CAT scan which revealed her shrunken liver tumors Francis asked if she was "partially cured." This was a perfect opportunity for either physician to explain the difference between partial remission, complete remission, and cure. Instead Dr. Keyes responded with "You are well on your way to a remission." Her response of, "Thank God, it's going away," made it clear that she didn't understand the situation. And by remaining silent, both doctors confirmed (in her mind) her belief. It also made the visit easier for them. And in robbing her of the truth they also robbed her of more time to process the information, come to terms with her prognosis, and take care of business. Groopman states that he realized in doing this he and Keyes had doubted their patient's ability to maintain hope, and their own ability as well.[11]

According to Dr. Groopman, some medical school courses are finally addressing the issue of how to give patients bad news, something not covered in the past but obviously needed.[12] He further describes how he finally learned from other physicians ways to honestly and gently share difficult truths while also extending hope.

Stage IV cancers, especially aggressive ones, often create situations in which there is no medical reason to hope for a physical cure. Doctors who view death as a personal failure may be at a loss about how to approach such patients. Certainly, I will admit that learning they are going to die is not something most patients want to hear (experience talking here). Words should be chosen carefully and conveyed with great sensitivity. Yet as Groopman states, "There is a middle ground where both truth and hope can reside." [13] This should be the physician's goal.

The way I see it the physician has two choices. He or she can share the diagnosis and prognosis as clearly as possible and tell the patient about any treatments or medical trials that might help. This means being fully honest about the odds. For example, the statement, "Statistically the odds may not be in your favor, but there is still a real chance this can help you," is realistic but also communicates hope. For most patients the diagnosis and related data may be overwhelming at first, which is why patients are often encouraged to bring a friend or family member along to take notes. In addition, the patient should be given key information in writing so they can read it again later when their mind is clearer.

What about the situation where the doctor doesn't believe the available treatments will provide any value to the patient at all or the risks of treatment far outweigh any potential benefits? I believe physicians should be fully honest with patients and tell them that their personal ethics prohibit offering the treatment in question. But palliative and hospice care should be strongly recommended because they are known to significantly increase quality and sometimes even quantity (length) of life.[14] If doctors have been building strong, caring, and trusting relationships with their patients, the patients will be far more likely to listen and follow this advice rather than jumping to the conclusion that their doctors are giving up on them.

Regardless of what decisions patients make physicians should inquire about their patients' hopes. There are always reasons for hope and things to hope for. If doctors have attempted, over time, to get to know their patients, they can learn what is most important to them (patients) and find ways to help them fulfill their hopes.

Of the many books I've recently read, two of my favorites are Being Mortal and Using the Power of Hope to Cope with Dying because they both do an excellent job of describing how physicians and other caregivers can help terminally ill patients identify and clarify realistic hopes and goals for themselves.[15, 16] Furthermore, they can explore with patients and family members how these hopes can be realized, even as their patients' health declines. Even patients who are resistant to such conversations may come around eventually. Such conversations can help them make sure they include or avoid things they feel strongly about, such as whether they want to die at home, be coded, be on a mechanical ventilator, have artificial nutrition, and so on. Further, it will help prompt them to have the hard but important conversations with their families about what they want. I know from personal experience how painfully difficult it is to make decisions for a loved one who can no longer speak for himself. One of the greatest gifts a patient can give to their loved ones (though nobody wants to discuss it at the time) is to complete a living will and make sure their family knows their wishes. It can make a painful and traumatic time, less painful and less traumatic (once again, experience talking here).

Even patients with very little time, can be helped to achieve some of their hopes and goals in their remaining days. Recall the account of Maria, described in the Introduction. From diagnosis to death, she lived only sixteen days. Most people might consider so little time inadequate to absorb the diagnosis much less identify and achieve any goals. Yet thanks to the support of loving friends, she was able to do both.

Chapter 11: Notes

1. George Bernard Shaw, "Brainy Quotes Home" George Bernard Shaw Quotes, http://www.brainyquote.com/quotes/authors/g/george_bernard_shaw.html. (Accessed 2/26/2017).

2. Honesty/Ethics in Professions, Website: http://www.gallup.com/poll/1654/Honesty-Ethics-Professions.aspx (accessed 4/1/2027).

3. Gawande, Atul. *Being Mortal: Medicine and What Matters in the End*. Metropolitian Books, Henry Holt and Co., New York, 2014. Kindle Edition. p. 167.

4. Walter Wangerin Jr. "Letters from the Land of Cancer." Copyright © 2010 by Walter Wangerin Jr. and/or Ruthanne M. Wangerin as Trustee of Trust No. 1. Zondervan. Kindle Edition. p. 32-33.

5. Ibid, p. 33.

6. Ibid, p. 33.

7. Ibid, p. 161.

8. Excellence Seminars International, www.excellenceseminars.com/ (Accessed 2/27/2017).

9. Groopman, Jerome. *The Anatomy of Hope: How People Prevail in the Face of Illness*. Random House Publishing Group. p. 30-33.

10. Ibid p. 50, Kindle location 641.

11. Ibid, p.50. Kindle location 234.

12. Ibid, p. 218. Kindle location 2473.

13. Ibid, p. 55. Kindle location 691.

14. Palliative Care Improves Quality of Life for Cancer Patients,

Presented by Massachusetts General Hospital Cancer Center, Boston © 2017 Metro Corp.

15. Chelsea Rice. Why Do Cancer Patients Like Menino Stop Treatment? October 24, 2014, Boston.com

16. See both books (below) on the Recommended Reading List

Groopman, Jerome. The Anatomy of Hope: How People Prevail in the Face of Illness Using the Power of Hope to Cope with Dying,

Gawande, Atul. Being Mortal: Medicine and What Matters in the End.

Chapter 12:
Pain

"Imagine smiling after a slap in the face. Then think of doing it twenty-four hours a day."[1]

Pain Management

The misuse and abuse of drugs is a real problem in this country and has sadly had a negative influence on the patient-physician relationship. Physicians who work in certain settings, such as emergency medicine may have more experience with patients who come in often and may be dubbed "frequent flyers." They are often believed to be seeking pain medication for inappropriate reasons and may be labeled "drug seekers" by healthcare providers. This sets the stage for a challenging and adversarial relationship between patients and healthcare providers. Once a patient has developed a reputation as a drug seeker, physicians become mistrusting of them and this influences their perception of whatever the patient says or does. As a result, even when the patient has a legitimate illness or injury and a justifiable reason for needing pain medication, physicians become reluctant to prescribe them.

Those who have never experienced severe pain, or unremitting pain severe enough to interfere with sleep and daily activities, can't appreciate the impact it has on quality of life. Pain of this sort, not adequately relieved by over-the-counter (OTC) analgesics, drives patients to seek relief. Not only does this sort of pain interfere with quality of life but it becomes physically, emotionally, and spiritually exhausting. Those who have experienced it become fearful of its continuation or its return. They not only fear the pain itself but also feel a loss of control over their own lives. All they want is relief. Enough relief that thoughts of pain move to the back of their mind rather than dominating their every thought. Enough relief to be able to sleep at night and to be active during the day. Unfortunately, all too often the expression of this fear is perceived as histrionics (being overly dramatic) by healthcare providers, which they interpret as drug-seeking behavior. If left untreated this pain can be a significant contributor to depression. For cancer patients it can become the last straw that impedes effective coping and robs them of the will to fight. They are already struggling to maintain hope and unrelieved pain may give them the reason they need to give up.

Until a reliable pain-o-meter is invented, doctors need to accept the fact that pain is subjective, and do what the pain management organizations state they should, which is to give patients the benefit of the doubt. Choose to believe them. Especially when the patient has cancer. Unless there is hard evidence to the contrary, all patients should be assumed to be relief seeking, not drug seeking. Consider the potential damage to the present and future patient-doctor relationship if the patient is assumed to be lying. Now compare that with the increased trust and rapport that is built when doctors choose to believe patients.

To make matters worse, physicians are monitored closely by certain regulatory agencies and may suffer punitive repercussions if thought to be over-prescribing. This is understandably a difficult position for physicians. Yet their ethical duty is to help their patients and they should not sacrifice their patients' needs due to such concerns.

Another issue which sometimes causes physicians to doubt their patients' veracity (truth-telling) is the subjective nature of pain and most other symptoms of discomfort. From the first day of medical school doctors are taught to rely heavily on objective (measurable, observable) data because it is easy to see and believe. They are much more comfortable with such information, especially when it relates to prescription of pain medication. If a patient has a fractured bone, a laceration (cut), a burn, or other obvious injury, doctors rarely hesitate to prescribe pain medication. But when the complaint is of a subjective nature—headache, back pain and the like—they are much more skeptical and often hesitate to write a prescription for opioids (narcotics) unless they can find some other corroborating evidence.

Historically, physicians have been extremely reluctant to prescribe opioid medications for patients with chronic pain. In fact, many doctors have simply refused. More recently some doctors have become slightly more willing but patients are monitored closely and even so, many doctors are still unwilling. Some physician concerns about giving opioids to the patient population with chronic pain are valid but many are not. In either case it is the subject matter for another book.

Traditionally doctors have been more willing to prescribe opioids for cancer patients, particularly those with terminal cancer. This is because physicians recognized their own limitations in what they had to offer such patients. They realized that if they could not provide a cure, there were only two things left. The first is to hopefully extend the length of the patient's life a bit longer through various types of treatment. The second is to hopefully improve the patient's quality of life, for whatever time they have left. This primarily includes the provision of pain relief and symptom management. Furthermore, if patients are going to die anyway, most physicians recognize the absurdity in worrying about issues of addiction. Therefore, when diagnosed with incurable cancer, most patients are encouraged by their doctors to take whatever pain medication they need and to not worry about related issues of tolerance, addiction, and dependency.

This happened to me. My primary care doctor, two radiation oncologists, and my oncologist all said the same thing, "If you need pain medication, take it." This was appropriate advice then and it still is. However, as time went by, I found myself experiencing something I had heard of, but could never comprehend; the reluctance of an oncologist to prescribe opioids to a terminally ill cancer patient. The thought had always baffled me. But now I find that it also frustrates and angers me. There is no justifiable reason for a patient with terminal cancer to ever suffer from unrelieved pain. This isn't just my opinion. Virtually every organization associated with pain research and pain management as well as other medical and nursing organizations all say the same thing. So why don't we practice what we preach?

JOURNAL JUNE 2011 FRUSTRATION WITH MY ONCOLOGIST

My oncologist keeps suggesting that my pain medication may be the cause of my fatigue. I know that opioids can cause sedation and drowsiness but only when someone first starts taking them. After a while the body develops tolerance to those side effects and they don't occur anymore. The only one that continues is constipation. I learned this during graduate school doing research for my thesis. I recently had a pharmacist recite this same information to me. My oncologist ought to know better. Either he does but hopes I do not, or he doesn't and really should. This was largely the topic of my graduate school research project, which is why I know. An oncologist should have more expertise in pain management than he seems to have. But then this is a point that became clear to me during my research.

Most physicians have exaggerated concerns about opioid side effects and inadequate concerns about the risks of non-opioid analgesics such as the millions of gastrointestinal (GI) bleeds and strokes caused by non-steroidal, anti-inflammatory drugs (NSAIDs) such as ibuprofen, naproxen, and aspirin. During my days as a hospital nurse I saw this over and over. Patients with pain are put on NSAIDs. Opioids are avoided because of perceived risks and concerns about addiction and side effects. As a result, they are often later admitted with serious, often life-threatening bleeding events. If the patient survives, they must make a tough decision between trying to live with their pain or risking another bleeding event.

Another key issue for doctors is the pressure they feel from regulatory groups, such as state medical boards and the Drug Enforcement Administration (DEA). Consequently, many become paranoid, fearing accusations of over-prescribing opioids to their patients, especially those with chronic, nonmalignant (non-cancer) pain.

JOURNAL AUGUST 2011
EXPERIMENT

Because my oncologist seemed so insistent in his belief that I should reduce my pain meds so I would experience more energy and less fatigue, I decided to experiment with them.

On two separate occasions I made a significant reduction in the amount I was taking for several days at a time. The result? I did not experience increased energy or decreased fatigue. But I did experience increased pain. The overall result was poorer quality of life. I described this to him more than once but he literally said nothing except, "Huh," and shrugged his shoulders. I could only assume he didn't believe me.

I believe medicine's failure to adequately address the physical, emotional, and spiritual pain of their patients is one of the key issues behind the assisted suicide movement. As long as patients have a quality of life that is acceptable to them, which always includes issues of comfort and symptom management, they rarely seek an escape. The notion of giving them medication to kill themselves is peddled as supporting their personal autonomy as well as their right to escape from pain. I'm all for autonomy. And I'm all for pain management. But I believe very few patients will make the choice to kill themselves if their healthcare providers give them good reasons not to. First and foremost, this includes pain and symptom management that is satisfactory to the patient. They should also be helped to identify hope and value in their lives, even at the end of life. If patients view their lives as meaningful and are provided with good physical, emotional, and spiritual care they are very unlikely to seek an escape. This might make the assisted suicide movement irrelevant.

The two most effective ways of doing this are to get patients involved in palliative care and hospice care. Sometimes patients or family members misunderstand the purpose of these services and assume it means patients are being asked to "give up" or that their physician is "giving up" on them. This isn't the case at all and virtually every patient that learns the truth about what palliative care and hospice offer choose one or both options at some point in their illness.

Palliative Care

According to the World Health Organization (WHO) "palliative care is an approach that improves the quality of life of patients and their families facing problems associated with life-threatening illness, through the prevention and relief of suffering by means of early identification and impeccable assessment and treatment of pain and other problems, physical, psychosocial and spiritual."[2]

Palliative care may be used at any point in the illness along with other therapies such as chemotherapy. It provides pain relief and symptom management and supports the patient in living the best quality of life possible. It provides support for the family during the patient's illness as well as bereavement following the patient's death. Palliative care philosophy views the dying process as a normal part of life, yet seeks to enhance quality of life for as long as the patient lives.

Hospice Care

Hospice care is a model of care designed specifically for patients with a terminal illness. It incorporates a team-oriented approach with a focus on high quality care including medical and nursing care, pain management, and emotional and spiritual care designed to meet individual patient's needs. Members of the team include physicians, nurses, home health aides, trained volunteers, therapists, social workers, and clergy as well as family members. At the heart of hospice and palliative care is the belief that each patient deserves to be treated with dignity and has the right to be pain-free.

A family member usually has healthcare power of attorney

(HCPOA) and helps make decisions for the patient. One or more family members provide primary, bedside care for the patient. Hospice staff visit regularly and provide additional care as needed. They are on-call twenty-four hours a day, seven days a week.

To learn more about hospice and palliative care see the National Hospice and Palliative Care Organization at their web site.[3] True stories about hospice patients and the care they receive are informative and inspirational. Some include Final Gifts, Final Journeys, Glimpses of Heaven, More Glimpses of Heaven, and One Foot in Heaven. These books are all written by hospice nurses with many years of experience. See my recommended reading list for these and other great books on related topics.

What's the Difference?

Since hospice and palliative care sound so similar some are confused between the two. So let me clarify. Anyone of any age, with any stage of any type of serious illness may qualify for palliative care. It does not depend on prognosis and you can have it at the same time you are having curative treatment. I would think the primary reason for seeking palliative care would be inadequate pain and symptom management. If the patient or concerned loved ones are not satisfied with the pain and symptom management currently being provided they should seek a palliative care consultation.

Hospice is a Medicare benefit that provides comfort care and end-of-life-care for terminally ill patients deemed to have less than six months to live. Those who choose hospice are no longer eligible to receive curative treatment. So using myself as an example, anytime I think I might benefit from palliative care I can ask for it. It doesn't matter if the doctor thinks I have six months or six years to live. It's all about improving quality of life for however long my life lasts. As long as I'm happy with my oncologist and my current level of care and current quality of life, I will probably not do this. But if or when any of those things change I will definitely consider it, especially if I haven't yet been deemed to be in my last six months of life. I would highly recommend the same to others, especially if you are less than satisfied with pain management and other quality-of-life issues that you currently have. Some doctors are very tuned in to quality-of-life issues and some are not, so don't wait for your doctor to suggest it. Be assertive and ask for it whenever you think you need it. The most important thing is that you get what you need. Don't worry about hurting the doctor's feelings. It's the doctor's job to take care of you, not the reverse. If that's not happening, then get a second opinion from another oncologist or get a palliative care consultation. There's just no good reason you should have to suffer in your last days. In fact, it's time to pull out the stops and make every day the best it can possibly be.

Regardless of whether I ever get palliative care involved with my case, I know for certain I will get hospice involved just as soon as I feel the "curative treatments" are no longer worth it. I have great respect for hospice and what they do. For me it's all about quality of life and making my last days the richest, fullest, most meaningful they can possibly be for myself and my loved ones. I know that hospice can help us do that.

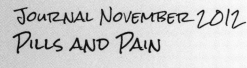

JOURNAL NOVEMBER 2012
PILLS AND PAIN

Pills, pills, pills. I take pills with my breakfast, pills with my lunch, pills with my dinner, pills between meals, and pills at bedtime. Some are scheduled and some are "as needed." It's surprising my stomach has any room left for food.

The same oncologist who told me to take pain pills "when I

need them" now seems to have changed his mind. His mixed messages are confusing and frustrating. Have I not died fast enough? Is my longevity making him nervous?

As a physician he gives "objective data" his attention and largely ignores the subjective which doesn't lend itself to observation or measurement. Since my scan results have been essentially unchanged he thinks my symptoms shouldn't have changed either. Yet I've gradually experienced a drop in energy level and a slow increase in pain. I'm grateful it hasn't been worse and that with medication, I've been relatively comfortable. However, the scans don't show what's going on in as much detail as he seems to think.

Pain and Opioids

The management of cancer-related pain has been widely accepted as an ethical duty of physicians.[4] Pain is defined in several ways. The International Association for the Study of Pain describes it as "an unpleasant emotional and sensory experience which may be related to tissue damage."[5] Another definition offered by nurse researchers McCaffrey and Beebe is, "Pain is whatever the experiencing person says it is, existing whenever the experiencing person says it does."[6] The second definition serves as a reminder that pain is subjective and known only to the experiencer. It does not lend itself to observation, testing, or measurement. One may make assumptions based upon the observation of certain behaviors. But assumptions are just that: assumptions. One cannot actually see pain. To really know what the individual feels one must ask and then listen.

Over the past twenty-five years or so, it has been widely acknowledged that the medical and nursing professions have done a very poor job of assessing and treating patients' pain of all types. It is estimated that twenty-five percent of cancer patients still die with unrelieved pain. This is totally unacceptable. Why does this happen? According to Weinstein and Janjan, pain remains untreated largely because of unfounded fears of addiction.[7] This is consistent with the survey findings of my graduate thesis and numerous other researchers.[8] The medical world has also been aware of this for at least twenty-five years, so again I ask "Why?" The answers, according to numerous medical experts, are poor pain management education in medical school, inadequate assessment of patients, reluctance of physicians to prescribe opioids, and regulatory barriers.[9] Even harder to understand is the fact that these trends are widely documented, including within cancer care centers where a third of the patients have been identified as having insufficient dosages of analgesics. If anyone should know better it's the experts in cancer care. So what gives?

My theory, which is well supported by copious data from various sources is that it is due to a combination of ignorance and fear. We've all heard for years how terrible the "drug problem" is and how we should just "say no" to drugs. But sadly there has never been a clear distinction between real drug abuse and the appropriate use of prescription medications for pain management. To add to the confusion, in recent years, certain prescription drugs (like oxycodone and fentanyl) have become preferred for abusers.

A few years before I had cancer, I heard of a politician who wanted to outlaw oxycodone because of this issue. It was a classic example of an inappropriate, knee-jerk response based on fear and ignorance. I was relieved that the idea didn't gain widespread acceptance. Most prescription medications are not inherently bad or good. They may be appropriate and work well for some people. And they may be inappropriate for others because they do not meet their needs or the risks outweigh the benefits. Oxycodone is an appropriate and effective medication for many people with cancer pain. It would be very sad for them to be deprived of it because other people choose to abuse it. We must take care not to punish the innocent for the crimes of the guilty.

People who take pain medication as well as any other substance for psychological effects are said to be misusing and potentially abusing them. Patients who take legally prescribed medication to manage their pain are not. I used to tell students in my pharmacology class that pain acts something like a "sponge" in the body. When taken for pain, opioids are "soaked up" by the pain-sponge leaving little or none to create psychological effects. However, opioids taken by someone with no pain are free to create psychological effects. So if a cancer patient is dosed with opioid analgesics, all they usually feel is better. They rarely have psychological effects, especially after the first few doses. Over time they may need larger doses because their pain has worsened or their body has developed tolerance. This is not addiction. In any case, when treating patients with cancer, especially terminal cancer, concerns about addiction or tolerance should never be a reason to withhold medication. Furthermore, all common side effects can usually be easily managed.

While most doctors are highly respected experts in their fields, most are not well-versed in the evaluation and treatment of pain. Furthermore, most have greatly exaggerated fears concerning potential side effects of respiratory depression, sedation, and the potential for addiction. Virtually all professional, medical information sources indicate that opioid treatment is appropriate for cancer patients, and fears of addiction should never be a reason for withholding medication. Yet many physicians, including some oncologists, are still afraid to prescribe opioids for their cancer patients.

Eventually I began to realize that my oncologist was one such doctor. As time went by, he commented more frequently that I ought to decrease my pain medications. Yet he failed to adequately explain why. One day I asked him directly what his main concern was and he replied that he simply wanted me to be at my best, mentally speaking, so I could enjoy a good quality of life. While this sounds like reasonable rationale, research indicates that it doesn't hold up. I knew that sedation resolves over time and shouldn't be a concern. I felt that he was not being fully honest. I explained that as a staff nurse I had administered pain medications to my patients, including cancer patients, thousands of times and could tell if they were becoming sedated. I did not see or feel those effects in myself. The pain medication simply allowed me to feel better so I could function; eat, sleep, and participate in other daily activities. This is in fact, the goal when medicating cancer patients; to increase quality of life by relieving pain and allowing them to function as fully as possible in their daily lives. Any good oncologist should know this.

Journal October 2013
Pain and Opioids

During my visit this month, without warning, my oncologist announced that he had reviewed my scans over the past year and didn't "believe the pain is that bad." Therefore, he decided to immediately cut my pain medication dosage in half with the goal of discontinuing it completely in the next several months. I was dumbfounded. I knew he had some concerns but I did not expect this. Virtually all professional sources regarding the treatment of pain in cancer patients are very clear in their recommendations that opioids should be used to treat cancer pain whenever necessary. As a nurse of some twenty-four years I also knew that it was never appropriate to withhold pain medication from a stage IV cancer patient, let alone suddenly cutting it in half.

So there I was, sitting in the exam room feeling like he had just called me a liar in front of my daughter, which meant he thought that I was just after the drugs. I was devastated. The one person in the world that I most needed to believe and support me had just disrespected me in the most awful manner possible. Furthermore, I felt trapped. If I tried to argue the reality of my pain and my need for medication, I feared appearing like the "drug seeker" he apparently believed me to be. If I stayed quiet and went along with his plan, I sacrificed myself, my personal integrity and my own truth. Additionally, I knew I was in for some hellish pain. I wanted to refuse what I knew to be an insane, unsafe and cruel plan. But I also wanted to be a good sport and seem reasonable, so I reluctantly agreed. What else could I do? As a patient I felt totally vulnerable and powerless. The following week was a nightmare.

I returned home committed to following my oncologist's plan. After all, I thought, "Maybe he is right. Maybe I will discover that I can get by with a reduced dose." In any case, I decided to give it my best shot and see what happened.

I was taking two different pain medications. One was a long-acting form that stayed in my system for a day or more, though it slowly decreased over time. The other was a short-acting form that peaked within one to two hours and was mostly gone after four to six hours. So between the two, it took a while for my blood levels to drop. I began the next morning by reducing both forms by half. That day, a Thursday, went ok. I had some increase in pain but it was bearable, so I thought, "Maybe this will be ok. Maybe I can do this." By Friday however, I began to have serious doubts. The pain intensified greatly throughout the day and by that night I was unable to sleep at all. By Saturday my pain was completely intolerable. I tried other pain management measures including distraction, careful stretching, massage, cold application, heat application, and positioning. But nothing helped. That night was a nightmare. By Sunday I was in tears with a pain rating of nine on the zero to ten pain scale. I felt quite literally as if someone were using a drill to bore a hole through the bones of my left sacrum. I could not imagine how I would feel if the medication was discontinued all together. That afternoon I finally gave in and took more of the medication I had on hand to equal my prior dosage.

My daughter and I had plans to leave town the next day and take her daughter to the zoo. I knew I would be miserable without adequate medication so I continued on my usual (prior) dosage and wrote a letter to my oncologist (Appendix A). I dropped it by his office before leaving town to make sure he received it that day. To my great relief he called me later in the week, thanked me for my "honesty" and promised to restore my medication dosage to its prior level. At my next office visit we would discuss the possibility of consulting a pain specialist. I felt like I had just experienced a stay of execution; immense relief for the short-term, but still dreading the final outcome.

I met with a physician pain specialist in November who tactfully stated that most doctors, including oncologists, are terrible at treating pain (which I already knew) and that suddenly cutting my medication dosage by half was totally inappropriate (which I also knew). He indicated that we could work toward reducing the opioid dosage but should do so slowly while we explore other forms of pain management. This made more sense to me and I left his office feeling some sense of relief.

Over the next several months we (Dr. Stevens, the pain special-ist, and I) experimented with increasing other medications I was already on while gradually reducing the opioids. In the end we succeeded in an approximate twenty-five percent dosage reduction which I am glad for. However, I knew my oncologist's idea of a total termination was absurd, and I failed to understand any rationale reason for it. Since I have stage IV cancer it is only a matter of time before the cancer spreads and pain worsens. It will eventually kill me and for anyone, much less an oncologist, to suggest I take no pain medication at all is crazy. Eventually I will need more rather than less.

Journal January 2014
Pain Management

I met with Dr. Stevens to discuss the medication reduc-tion plan and asked what he thought about it. He was quite tactful and said nothing disrespectful about the other doc-tors but did say since he has known me for many years he has zero concern about me misusing the meds. He acknowledged that we had "made progress" in the plan, saw no reason to further reduce the dosage and felt fine maintaining it at the current level. With his approval I also made an appointment to see a different oncologist. It was so refreshing to meet with someone who knows me, and trusts and believes me!

During February I met with Dr. Shell, a different oncologist in the same department, and found myself liking her very much. She seemed genuinely interested in my situation and actually listened when I answered her questions. She doubted I would ever get off all the pain medication, nor did she think I needed to. She agreed that quality of life issues matter most and felt it reasonable to maintain my current medication dose for the time being.

Journal May 2014
Pain

During the past few months I noticed a modest increase in my sacral pain. After my previous experience I was a bit anxious about reporting it, fearing I might not be believed. But being the caring professional that she is, Dr. Shell listened empathetically. She then ordered a new CT scan which revealed an extension of the sacral lesion (objective data!). I was half tempted to slip a copy of the report under my previous oncologist's door just to prove to him that I wasn't lying about my pain. But I knew that was childish so I resisted temptation. However, at Dr. Shell's suggestion I met with a radiation oncologist to see if further radiation might be helpful. I subsequently underwent two more weeks of radiation therapy for this new area of mets on my sacrum. It worked fairly well. I still have pain there but it is less severe and less frequent than before. I've still not needed to increase my medication dose. And a nice bonus was that I had no GI side effects this time. Yay!

Over the next year I did quite well pain-wise and needed no increase in medication. I still feel quite satisfied with Dr. Shell. She does not run on autopilot as my other oncologist seemed to and asks different questions each time, delving into different aspects of my condition and my life. She is an empathetic listener and is open to ideas or suggestions that might improve my quality of life.

JOURNAL JUNE 2015
REFLECTIONS OVER THE PAST TWO YEARS

I expect it's obvious that I was quite frustrated with my first oncologist and his pain management skills (or lack thereof). As I reflect on the entire experience I am reminded that most cancer patients are not medical professionals. They don't speak the language and have little or no medical education. I feel especially badly for the frail elderly who are a part of the generation that never questioned their doctor's actions. The era when physicians were deemed to be nearly god-like and incapable of mistakes. How many such patients are out there suffering right now because they don't know how to question their doctor and advocate for themselves? Being a patient is a difficult, scary and vulnerable place to be, regardless of who you are. We depend on our healthcare providers to be caring, empathetic, and informed. And we need them to be more concerned about our agendas than their own. I fear this issue might explain why twenty-five percent of cancer patients still die in pain.

Chapter 12 Notes

1. Markus Zusak. *The Book Thief.* Alfred A. Knopf publisher, New York, 2005.

2. Definition of palliative care found at this World Health Organization website: WHO who.int/cancer/palliative/definition/en/ (accessd 4/1/2017).

3. Definition of hospice care can be found at this website: nhpco. org/about/hospice-care (accessed 3/27/2017).

4. Sandra H. Johnson, JK, LLM. "Legal and Ethical Perspectives on Pain Management, Anesthesia & Analgesia." July 2007-Volume 105 Issue 1. pp 5-7.

   Fr. Peter A. Clark, S.J., Ph.D., Ethical Implications of Pain Management, July-August 2002, Catholic Health Association of the U.S.

   Salma Amin Rattini, Ethical Perspective of Cancer Pain Management, June 29, 2015, International Journal of Nursing Education.

5. https://en.wikipedia.org/wiki/International_Association_for_the_Study_of_Pain (Accessed 5/28/2017).

6. McCaffery, Margo, and Alexandra Beebe. *Pain: Clinical Manual for Nursing Practice.* C. V. Mosby, St. Louis, 1989.

7. Sharon M. Weinstein MD, FAAHPM and Nora Janjan, MD, MPSA, MBA, June 1, 2015, Management of Pain, Cancer Network.

8. Huck, Sharon., Gonzaga University, Spokane WA, Graduate Thesis, 1994.

9. Ibid, Weinstein and Janjan.

Chapter 13
Reconciliation

"Peace is not absence of conflict,
it is the ability to handle conflict by peaceful means."[1]

Most people nearing death realize they have a certain amount of "unfinished business" they need to attend to. Among other things, this often includes reconciliation in certain relationships. Sometimes there is simply another, "I love you," to be said. But in other cases there has been serious estrangement for a period of time and the individual doesn't want to die without making some attempt to mend fences and heal old wounds.

As a nurse I've seen families come together around a loved one's bed during the last days or hours of their life. I've seen the situation bring out the worst and the best in them. Sometimes there is anger, resentment and a life time of dysfunction. And sometimes there is no reconciliation and no healing. People sometimes remain stuck in the past and stuck in their emotional stuff, refusing to forgive and missing their last opportunity to make peace.

Other times I've seen amazing healing occur in relationships. Loved ones who'd been estranged, sometimes for years, finally remembering that they love one another. Recognizing that their relationships are more important than their grudges. It's amazing how the impending death of a loved one can bring perspective—if we let it. Even though it's a sad, sometimes tragic situation, it can also be an amazing time of love, forgiveness, healing, and reconciliation. It is such an awesome gift that loved ones can give to one another—if they are willing.

As a nurse I occasionally saw cases in which I believed reconciliation was needed. But my first duty was always to the patient, to act as his or her advocate. So I could make suggestions and help facilitate communication and visitation if needed. But I could not force it and I had to maintain the confidentiality of my patient's condition and medical history. So sometimes it was easy and quite gratifying to play my role. And at other times it left me sad and frustrated. One such patient, many years ago, was one of my first AIDs patients. He was in his fifties, didn't have long to live and seemed quite alone without any visitors at all. As we became better acquainted I gently asked if he had any family or friends he would like me to call. He shared that he had one adult son from whom he'd been estranged for many years. Apparently when he'd come out and let others know that he was gay, his son hadn't taken it well. He didn't share the details but did say that they hadn't spoken in many years. He said his son was angry and ashamed of him and had never forgiven him. Now that he was dying he did not want his son to know and did not want him to be contacted.

I tried to change his mind but was not successful. So all I could do was try to provide good nursing care and be an empathetic listener when he felt like talking. It didn't feel like enough and I always wondered if his son had any regrets when he got word of his father's death. I know that words can sometimes wound deeply and some relationships are beyond repair but I've also found that when death is imminent, most people recognize what is most important and are willing to put old quarrels aside and let love rule. At least I like to think so.

Journal August 2010
An Example of Reconciliation

A few weeks ago I accidentally made a phone call to a person by the name of Cindi. I had disliked her in the past because of emotional wounds I believed she had inflicted on my family, especially my children. I will say that God certainly has an interesting sense of humor and somehow He knew that my heart was in a place where I was ready to have a conversation with her. So I somehow managed to misdial my phone that day and instead of hearing the voice of the person I meant to call, to my great surprise I heard Cindi's voice mail pick up. In a sort of knee-jerk response, I hit the disconnect button and stood there totally baffled as to how I had managed to call her. I was sure her number had been deleted from my phone years before. As I was pondering the matter my phone rang and I saw her name on the caller ID. I quickly realized that being a businesswoman, of course she didn't want to miss a call. So I answered the phone and listened to her identify herself. At that point the entire thing struck me as funny and I started laughing. I proceeded to identify myself and explained to her what had happened. She had heard news of my cancer diagnosis and reached out to me in a way I did not expect, offering help and support. As it turned out, we chatted for quite a while that day and ended the conversation on very good terms. After I hung up the phone, the word that hit me was reconciliation. Not just forgiveness but something more. I cannot tell you how good it felt and as impossible as it once seemed, I now count this person as a friend. I've seen her socially since then and it has been a good thing. I think we both needed the healing that occurred. I know I did.

Reconciliation with my Father

I had not been in touch with my father for over twenty-five years. It's a lengthy and unpleasant story that touches on the lives of many people whom I care deeply about. Initially I felt reluctant to share it for fear of adding to the hurt that's already been inflicted. Yet I realized that telling the story of reconciliation in my life would be incomplete without this part. Further, it is unrealistic to think that reconciliation always works in every situation. Love doesn't always win out, as much as we might wish that it did. This isn't a fairly-tale after all. It's a true tale about a real life. This means I must share some of the ugliness along with the beauty.

As a small girl I thought my daddy was perfect. And the truth is that he did have some wonderful qualities. After all, none of us is entirely good or bad, but a mixture of the two. He was warm and affectionate and unlike the daddies of some of my friends, he actually enjoyed spending time with his children. He liked to include us in whatever he was doing and was a natural teacher. With him we learned a bit of geology because we were a family of rock hounds. It was impossible not to be, given that my grandparents lived on top of a petrified forest. There we learned to cut and polish the rocks to bring out their natural beauty. At their farm and ours, Dad taught us a great deal about animals, something I've always been grateful for. At various times we owned beef cattle, dairy cattle, chickens, pigs, ducks, peacocks, rabbits, a horse, cats, dogs and mink (yes those furry critters they make coats out of). I learned how to behave around animals so as to not startle or frighten them. When they were ill or injured I learned to help care for them. I fed orphaned calves formula through a bucket with a large nipple on it, and piglets from an animal baby bottle. Over time we collected a small gang of outcasts and misfits that others would have euthanized. But my siblings and I wanted to adopt and care for them and our dad supported us in doing so. At one point we had a "runt" arthritic pig named Wilbur, an arthritic rooster named Ben, and a blind calf named Donde. There were too many cats over the years to remember them all. But I do recall Mr. White the muscular hunter and consummate farm cat. Once, while moving bales of hay in the barn, my dad and my brother Rick saw him catch three mice at once; one with his mouth and one with each front paw. We also learned to help grow and harvest various crops and grew up with a great appreciation for nature.

We each had a unique relationship with our dad. One of my favorite things was watching him shave. I loved watching him mix up the shave soap in its cup, and brush it on his face and neck leaving him all foamy. The best part came next as he shaved it off strip by strip. There was something magical about how his whiskers disappeared each time, leaving his face fresh, shiny, and smooth. Eventually I developed my own routine which allowed me to copy him. I'd climb on a chair so I could look into the mirror next to him. After he finished with the soap I would take a turn spreading it over my face. Then I'd use the back of a comb to "shave" it off and end up with a face that was clean and smooth, just like his.

Dad was a smoker. In those early days we didn't realize how damaging it was to our bodies. I just knew that I enjoyed the ritual of watching him strike a match, light his cigarette, inhale, and then blow out the first puff of smoke. There was something about the smell of a freshly lit cigarette that I loved. I still do. These days I am thoroughly versed in the many destructive qualities of cigarettes and you'd have to search long and hard to find someone more anti-smoking than me. Yet I still love that smell. But it only lasted for the first puff or two. Then the magic was lost and it turned into yucky, stale smoke.

As I reflect back over my childhood, now from the perspective of an adult and mother, I cringe at some of the ill-advised decisions my father made. He loved having us with him, which was great, but he often lacked the good judgment one would expect of an adult. I knew I could always get a "yes" from him, so if I wanted a snack before dinner I would ask him. That put Mom in the unwanted position of being the disciplinarian and responsible parent who made me put the snack away. Small situations like that were a daily occurrence. But they weren't all small. One day he made the horrific decision to allow my siblings and I (all five of us approximate ages five through twelve) to climb aboard the tractor with him and ride from our home across town and out into the country where my grandparents farm was located; approximately five to ten miles. If you've ever seen a tractor you know there is just one seat. How we each found a place to stand and hold on without falling off throughout the entire journey amazes me. I think our angels were looking out for us that day. You may understand the anxiety and worry our mother felt. By the time she caught up with us at the farm she was a jumble of nerves in a puddle of tears. So what sort of comfort and reassurance did she receive from her loving husband and his parents? Uh, none. They spent the next hour berating and belittling her about "making a big deal out of nothing." As they all ganged up on our mom, my siblings and I could only stand by feeling guilty and sorry for her. We were just children but we knew who was right and who was wrong. That was the first time I recall beginning to hate my grandad. He was so mean to my mom and treated her terribly. At times my dad joined in and at others he simply stood back and watched. But he never stood up for her.

There are many more family tales, some good, some not. But to the heart of the matter of why I hadn't spoken to him for twenty-five years . . . .

It was 1977 and I was engaged to be married in early November. Like many young brides I wanted my father to walk me down the aisle. By this time, I was twenty-one years old and well aware that my father was not perfect. But he was still my dad and I still loved him in spite of his flaws. He was scheduled to drive north with his third wife and three stepdaughters to join us for the wedding. Then just three days before hand he called with the news that he would be traveling alone. Explaining the reason and events around this decision would require an entire book of its own. But the short story is that he had been arrested in late spring of that year for molesting several of the children in his third grade class. Of course he pleaded innocent and being a consummate liar as most pedophiles are, he was able to tell fairly believable versions of his side of the story. In my heart, I think I knew he was guilty from the start, but I wanted so badly to believe in his innocence. However, when confronted with a lie detector test, he finally crumbled and confessed to the crime. He even explained it all in a letter he wrote to my sister. To make matters even worse than they already were, he had been molesting his stepdaughters as well. When confronted with this news I felt sick but was also in a state of shock and didn't know how to respond. To say I was disappointed in him would be a huge understatement. I hated what he had done. Yet nothing would change the fact that he was still my father. I felt like my heart and mind were split. He would always remain the daddy of my childhood and on some level I still loved him. But I didn't know how to reconcile this with the monster he had become; someone who could do such horrendous things to innocent children. I knew all too well the sort of pain and injury inflicted on those young girls and I felt so badly for them. Over the next five years he was on probation, underwent mandatory counseling (which had no effect), and made some efforts to get his life back together. Somewhere along the way he moved to the area where I lived which meant I saw him more often than before. It was hard enough as his daughter trying to determine if I could maintain a relationship with him. But then my own family began to grow and I quickly realized that I wasn't comfortable having him around my children. There were a few visits, supervised closely by me. In the meantime I tried to find my footing to see if we could renegotiate some sort of father-daughter relationship. But it just never worked. Even the most basic conversations turned into bizarre events in which he would act the victim and trash-talk whomever it was this time who had attacked, betrayed, or otherwise treated him poorly. If I sympathized with him, I sacrificed my own integrity because I knew him well enough by then to know that his version of the story held little truth. But if I challenged him with facts or any semblance of reality he became angry and argumentative, and attacked my credibility. It was a no-win situation so I usually remained silent which also felt wrong. I was greatly relieved the day he announced he was moving back south to his previous home. After that our contact quickly dwindled to rare phone calls, then to annual Christmas cards and then eventually to nothing.

As I've been coping with cancer and trying to learn whatever lessons God has for me I kept feeling the need to make some sort of attempt at reconciliation. This was not the first time. I'd made numerous efforts in the distant past but I was never able to have a relationship with him that worked for both of us. It felt like unfinished business and I couldn't seem to let it go. Or maybe it wouldn't let go of me. I'm not really sure. Either way I felt compelled to give it one last try, so I composed a letter to him in which I told him of my illness and some of the spiritual lessons I'd been learning; especially those related to trust, gratitude, and forgiveness.

I mentioned that I've come to believe that one of the reasons he was meant to be my father was so that I could learn about forgiveness. I also mentioned that there is something about facing my own impending death that has been helping me finally get my priorities into place and I realized that I have no desire to hold onto anger, grudges, or other forms of negativity. Perhaps he didn't take this well, but it was and is my truth.

I was writing to tell him that I had forgiven him for the insanely hurtful things he'd done over many years to our family and members of our community. I also mentioned the idea of some form of reconciliation.

Journal July 2010
So much for reconciliation

I received a reply today from Dad. I suppose it was foolish of me to hope that he might have changed at all. It was a bizarre, five-page letter filled with venomous accusations around a bizarrely re-invented history that in no way resembled actual events. He described a litany of wounds my siblings, my mother, and I had supposedly inflicted on him, conspiracy-style. After all these years he is angrier than ever which is odd given that he was the one that hurt others. But as usual he excels at playing the victim and has forgotten that I was there too. I remember what happened. He made no comments about what I'm going through health-wise or what Rob went through (or why he didn't bother to come to the hospital when Rob was dying). In fact, he really didn't comment on anything I said in my letter other than to say he was sure I'd "be fine." Furthermore, he went on and on about how he has found a new family and how much they trust him (in a manner we did not) and how they are his true family now so we had better not ask him to choose because he will choose them every time. One of the many sad things about this is that I've heard it all before. He has invented new families several times over the years and loves to point out how much more they trust him than we ever did and how he will always pick them over us. Not surprisingly, none of us has ever asked him to choose. But he loves to be dramatic.

I might feel angry if I had the energy, so maybe it's a good thing I don't. I suppose this is a confirmation of how extremely dysfunctional he is and how pointless it would be to try to have any sort of relationship with him. However, I'm glad I wrote because it was therapeutic for me to do so, and though we didn't achieve true reconciliation I do feel a sense of peace and closure that I didn't before. Sometimes in life, there are people we are just not meant to have relationships with.

Journal July 2010
My Brother's Response

Since I was upset upon first receiving the letter from Dad, I wrote to two people who I knew could understand, my sister Stephenie and my younger brother Roger. I sent each of them copies of both letters; mine and my father's. Roger's response (below) was insightful and comforting.

"Probably most people learn and grow over the years and through experience. But some don't. Our earthly father is in the second category. Your letter, though written to him, is valuable to me. I respect and cherish your thoughts and feelings and inspirations. Remember that the swine behaving badly does not make the pearls cast before them any less pearly. Tromping and more endless tromping and still the pearls and gems remain what they are. Beautiful!

Fortunately, our heavenly Father does not forget His children. We are His. And He is ours. And that doesn't change. I'm very grateful that my sisters and brothers are my sisters and brothers in the eternal sense. That makes all the difference."

I decided not to reply to my father. I'd been there before and knew it was pointless. I have been at peace about the issue since. I feel no further inclination or need to communicate with him. I made my attempt at reconciliation and I think maybe that was all God was asking of me.

Daily Reconciliation

Recently I realized another reason God is having me live with my son and his wife. As we live together and do the best we can to support one another, miscommunication and conflict are inevitable. Therefore, reconciliation is something that must be revisited frequently, even daily. This is true for any healthy relationship. So if we value them we must practice reconciliation. This requires some degree of humility, willingness to apologize and admit to mistakes, as well as asking and receiving forgiveness. For any of this to work all parties must value the relationship over their need to be "right" and "win" arguments.

Mother-Son Reconciliation

I recently had a conversation with Brad about something that had weighed on my heart since he was a boy of eight. When we divorced his dad insisted we let Brad choose with whom he wanted to live. I made the mistake of agreeing and immediately realized what a horrific mistake it was. We had placed him right in the middle and forced him to choose between his mother and father. Emotionally speaking, it's one of the worst things parents can do to a child. My heart still breaks when I recall how torn he was by this decision. And though he chose his father, so his "dad wouldn't be alone" what hurt me the most was the agony we had put him through. I told him how I deeply regretted our actions back then and said if I had a chance to go back and change one thing in my life that would be it. In any case God has an amazing way of making lemonade out of our lemons. In the same conversation Brad shared how he had felt God working in his life a few years ago. As a result, he had reflected upon that painful time in his life and felt God had prepared him for our conversation this day. So even though I felt undeserving of Brad's forgiveness, he offered it anyway. He said he had found a way to learn and grow from it all in spite of our screw-up. He has grown into such an amazing man and I am so honored to be his mother. And so grateful.

Reconciliation with Ex-husband(s)

When I was a young, naïve bride of twenty-one I never dreamed I would end up divorced once, much less twice. After all these years it still feels difficult to admit to. Each time my marriage ended I felt in some ways like a failure and knew I had let many people down. However, it was a tremendous journey of learning and growth. And one of the very good things that came from it is that I learned a great deal about reconciliation. That's not to say that we reconciled the marriage(s) but we did learn to forgive, let go of animosity, and become friends. Based on my own observations of other divorced couples, I believe this is rather uncommon. I've seen so many couples who, even after many years, still feel anger, hostility, and resentment toward one another. In my opinion such negativity serves no useful purpose and continues to hurt both parties as well as children and other family members.

I will admit it took some time, but I'm pleased to say that I developed friendly, pleasant, and amiable relationships with both of my exes. This has been especially beneficial with the father of my children. Regardless how much time passes, he will always be their father and, married or not, we will always be family. We both love our children and grandchildren and want only the best for them. And we both want to continue being involved in their lives. Keeping score and taking turns may be the best that some can achieve but such situations remain stressful and unpleasant for everyone.

After our marriage ended, my first ex-husband and I both eventually married again. Sadly, those marriages did not last. Yet after so many years we both found ourselves in a place where we no longer felt animosity toward each other and wanted to gain a better understanding of what had contributed to the demise of our marriage. So, after years of barely speaking, we met for a lunch that turned into a five-hour conversation. We covered a lot of ground, answered questions, and resolved many issues. Since then, we've had other conversations, sometimes about our history but mostly about our children. We've achieved a point of being quite comfortable with each other, and now we both join our children and grandchildren for holidays, birthdays, occasional dinners, and our grandchildren's school and sport events. We even went on a family vacation together last year with all the kids and grandkids and had a great time. We are not "back together" in a romantic sense, but we have a comfortable friendship and are able to talk about most things. The healing that's occurred between us and within our entire family feels wonderful.

Because we didn't have any mutual kids, I see much less of my second ex-husband, who has moved to another city, but we are on friendly terms and communicate occasionally via e-mail and Facebook, and we wish only the best for each other. A real bonus is that I've maintained a good relationship with his daughters and their mother (his first wife) and will always consider them family. It's funny where life takes us. And though things don't always turn out the way we plan, life can still be very good.

Reconciliation with Self

Sometimes the person we are most reluctant to forgive is ourselves. I touched on my own reluctance in the story above about Brad. As a mother I felt so guilty about the wound we had inflicted on him and knew I'd never be able to forgive myself if he didn't forgive me first. I didn't seek his forgiveness for many years, because I felt I didn't deserve it, but eventually I broached the subject because I wanted him to know how deeply I regretted it, whether he ever chose to forgive me or not. As it turned out, he did forgive me— something not everyone would do under such circumstances. So then I was able to finally forgive myself. It can still bother me if I let it. But when such thoughts come to mind I remind myself of all Jesus went through so that we can all be forgiven. Then I remind myself of the gift of love and forgiveness my son offered me. With all of this in mind I realized that if I didn't accept forgiveness from both of them it would be like disrespecting the amazing gifts they were handing me.

Most people struggle to some degree with the reluctance or inability to forgive. Sometimes they resist forgiving others. Sometimes they resist forgiving themselves. One of the patients whom Dr. John Lerma interviewed suggested that if we don't do the work of self-forgiveness now, it will take us longer to feel comfortable in heaven. Another patient in the same book advises us to not wait until we are on our deathbed to work out our issues. She says learning to love ourselves is the key to being able to love others and that we will feel less overwhelmed on our deathbeds if we work out our issues today. As we come to understand and accept ourselves we are better able to love ourselves and then better able to love others. As this occurs she believes it will help us to resolve much of the bigotry and hatred in the world. It makes sense to me.

I'm not sure about how comfortable I will or won't feel in heaven when I first get there but I can see where it is good for personal emotional health and spiritual well-being to gain forgiveness from anyone I have wronged, including myself. I know that therapists make entire careers helping people with such things so it must be worthwhile. Furthermore, I know from experience that my feelings about myself do impact my feelings about other people.

The Anatomy of Reconciliation

Some may be baffled by my ability to reconcile with my ex-husbands and even their past or present wives. Some may think, "Well that's fine for you but you don't know what she did to me." That may be true but let me assure you that there was plenty of drama, emotional injury, pain, and selfishness to go around. Reconciliation did not come easily, or without a tremendous amount of work. But I decided that I had no wish to carry the associated pain and anger with me indefinitely and wanted to heal. I knew I had developed the necessary tools in my earlier life to work through it all. And most importantly, I had a clear vision of the results I wanted to create. I wanted a good life with those I loved, unhindered by the angst and anger that holding grudges would cause. I was willing to admit that this goal was more important to me than any wounds or hurt feelings I might wish to hold on to. This clarity helped me to let it all go.

Reconciliation is an important consideration for anyone facing a terminal illness. And it brings peace. Peace of mind but maybe more importantly peace of heart. Forgiving and being forgiven— both emotionally and spiritually—are such a healing thing.

So I share parts of my own journey to any who will listen with the goal of encouraging you to get your priorities in order. Don't let old grudges and disputes and your need to be right cheat you and others of the healing and joy that reconciliation can bring.

Most people have at least one relationship in their life that needs reconciliation. If you are such a person, but don't know where to start, you might try some or all of the following.

- Identify what about the relationship does and does not work for you.
- Be assertive in reaching out yet willing to make yourself vulnerable.
- Share your major motivation (like you want this person in your life).
- Avoid becoming defensive.
- Share pain without expressing blame.
- Express love, seek and extend forgiveness.

Bringing people together, sometimes across great distances, to gather at the bedside of a dying loved one can provide meaningful opportunities for reconciliation. As friends and family come together, individuals who have been estranged may find that old issues resurface. Willingness to let go of old grudges and to seek healing of relationships can go a long way toward fostering family unity and promote healing of old wounds. Furthermore, it can be an important step in the process of facilitating a peaceful death for the ill person.

Chapter 13 Notes

1. Ronald Reagan. BrainyQuote.com, Xplore Inc, 2017. https://www.brainyquote.com/quotes/quotes/r/ronaldreag169550.html (Accessed 5/29/2017).

Chapter 14
Depression

"Depression is the most unpleasant thing I have ever experienced. . . . It is that absence of being able to envisage that you will ever be cheerful again. The absence of hope. That very deadened feeling, which is so very different from feeling sad. Sad hurts but it's a healthy feeling. It is a necessary thing to feel. Depression is very different." [1]

Is depression a natural part of the dying process? I used to think it was probably unavoidable as I noticed that most of my terminally ill patients were on antidepressants. Eventually I learned there is no rule that dictates such patients must be given antidepressants. Rather, I believe the practice is the result of how most health care providers think in a society where death is feared and largely denied. In our culture, death is something of a taboo subject and most doctors view it as an enemy to be conquered. When patients die, even expectedly, most physicians view it as a personal failure. Even oncologists, who should know better, sometimes struggle with this. I've also learned that antidepressants are used to treat a number of things in addition to depression. Examples include hot flashes, insomnia, and neurogenic (nerve) pain.

Is Depression to Be Expected?

I found it interesting that I never felt the anger that one hears about and thus far have not experienced any significant depression. Yes, I've felt quite sad at times and may cry sometimes but it never lasts long, especially when I remember to focus on gratitude. I've wondered why I didn't struggle more with issues of denial, anger and depression. I've seen others overwhelmed by them. I'd like to think it's because I'm such a mentally healthy and "together" person, but that seems rather arrogant. It made a bit more sense to me when I read Dying Well, an excellent book which I highly recommend.[2] In it the author points out the common, but incorrect belief that terminal illness and depression always go together. Instead he describes a "normal grief reaction" that is quite different from clinical depression. In this reaction people may feel normal sadness and depressed mood that can be treated, if need be, with nonmedical care. He further states that an individual's susceptibility is related more to biology, temperament, heredity, and self-image than to their current health situation.[3] Correctly identifying patients with severe clinical depression requires careful evaluation, since those with metastatic cancer may develop side effects from the cancer or its treatment that can mimic those of severe depression (anorexia, weight loss, sleep disruption, and fatigue).[4] Therefore, first impressions might be misleading and cause physicians to assume patients are depressed when they are not.

An estimated fifteen to fifty percent of cancer patients are thought to have some form of depression, while only five to twenty percet struggle with severe depression.[5] So it seems I am not as unique as I first thought but it's good to know that depression isn't a given.

Major Depressive Disorder

Major depressive disorder or clinical depression is a serious form of depression that should be treated. According to the Mayo Clinic, it affects how a person feels, acts and thinks and can cause various physical and emotional problems.[6] Depressed people may have difficulty performing regular daily activities, are often irritable, and struggle with memory, concentration, and feelings of hopelessness. They may need long term treatment and usually respond best with a combination of medication and psychological counseling.[7]

My friend Grace, a nurse who specializes in mental health issues, noticed some subtle changes in my behavior since my diagnosis. I wasn't aware of it until she pointed it out but I was grateful for her concern. Essentially she wondered whether I was experiencing serious depression or just some temporary withdrawal as I pondered my mortality. Her question prompted me to consider the subject both on a general and a personal level.

Having recently undergone chemotherapy and radiation, I had been suffering from anorexia, weight loss, sleep disruption, and fatigue, so my overall energy level was quite low. Therefore I understood how others might have misinterpreted this as depression. And these things certainly reduced my activity level which could have, once again, been interpreted as depression. I expect some people do experience both so the issue can be confusing.

I had noticed that I was much more introspective and wrestled with many conflicting thoughts and feelings. It felt impossible to describe to one who hasn't been there. I wasn't done living and was still enjoying many things about my life—and I wanted to continue living the best quality life I could for whatever time I had left. At the same time, I needed to come to grips with my mortality in a real way that I never had to before. This meant that I pondered what my life was going to be like as my physical health and energy continue to decline. I also pondered what my healthcare needs would be and worried about the loss of independence that may be involved. Then there were the questions about what my death would be like and the huge questions about what follows. I was also busy doing what I could to "take care of business" to ease the pain of my passing for my family—to whatever extent I could. In a weird way, it feels a bit like having a foot in both worlds. I think of someone anticipating a move. One foot still in the here and now and one (sort of) in the world to come. It's very difficult to describe the indescribable. I think that is one reason I appreciate the book Final Gifts so much. The authors do a nice job of at least partially describing what the journey is like for people who are dying. Granted I am not dying yet and (hopefully) am still very early on in that journey, yet I could still relate to many of the things they described. I know that sometimes people do become depressed. But I understand now better than I have before, the need to turn inward and reflect on one's life and reexamine priorities.

This almost feels like a developmental stage to me. Psychologists have done a pretty good job of analyzing and understanding the developmental stages that people go through early in their lives. But I think few understand the ones people go through near the end of life. Perhaps thinking about it feels too scary and reminds them of their own mortality. Furthermore, we can all relate to the earlier stages in life because we've all been through them. However, most people that do the research and writing, have not yet been through the latter stages and thus, cannot relate to them. I've always thought that healthcare providers are way too quick to assume people are depressed when perhaps they are simply taking time and energy to reflect on life and death or in some cases have achieved a state of full acceptance of their impending death. Most people can't seem to understand or accept that this might be a good and healthy thing—therefore the assumption is made that the person is depressed. And then physicians haven't a clue what to do about it so they write prescriptions for anti-depressants.

I actually feel that I'm in a pretty good place emotionally speaking and it's good to know I have a great support system. But it is an odd journey to be on and I'm sort of figuring it out as I go along. That's not to say that depression might not be an issue for me in the future, but it isn't now.

Withdrawal

I've heard that withdrawal is a normal behavior for people who are terminally ill. I understand this better now. There is a certain amount of emotional and spiritual work required to prepare for death. It's not that I'm eager to go but I accept that it is inevitable and so I'm trying to deal with it the best that I can. Then there's all of the misery that accompanies a worsening physical condition and this leaves me very little physical and emotional energy for anything else. Sometimes the only thing I feel like doing is curling up with a pillow and blanket and sleeping. But then I think about how limited my time with my family is, and how I need to make the most of it. I don't want to waste it all sleeping.

Various terms are used for the process in which cancer patients experience a sort of emotional distance or numbness from the immediate situation. This allows us to think about it without feeling emotionally overwhelmed. The terms detachment and withdrawal are often used. But I believe a more accurate term is introspection which literally means "a reflective looking inward; an examination of one's own thoughts and feelings."[8] The synonyms of self-analysis or soul-searching may be more familiar to most people.

Whatever you prefer to call it, this is a very normal process and the patient will most likely experience it at some point in time; possibly more than once. With the knowledge that one's life is approaching its end, it's quite normal for people to reflect back over their lives and wonder if they've been meaningful. I've done this extensively at various times and wondered whether I had made the most of my life. In fact, given a terminal diagnosis, I would be a bit worried about the person who doesn't do some introspection. When a person is in an introspective mode they may be quieter and appear more serious than usual. Others might mistake this for depression. However, the two are really quite different. So don't make the mistake of assuming that all terminally ill people are or will be seriously depressed, just know that it's a possibility. If depression is suspected, the best course of action is to have the individual evaluated and if necessary, treated by a mental health expert. Dealing with a fatal illness is difficult enough without needlessly suffering from depression.

Chapter 14 Notes

1. https://www.goodreads.com/quotes/388617-depression-is-the-most-unpleasant-thing-i-have-ever-experienced   (Accessed 5/29/2017).

2. Ira Byock. *Dying Well: The Prospect for Growth at the End of Life*. Riverhead books, New York, 1997. p. 101.

3. Dialogues Clin Neurosci. 2011 Mar; 13(1): 101–108. Depression and End-of-life Care for Patients with Cancer;

4. Ira Byock, MD. *Dying Well*. "Depression and End-of-life Care for Patients with Cancer to distinguish between normal grief reactions and clinical depression." Penguin Publishing Group. p. 101.

5. Ibid

6. Mayo clinic.org www.mayoclinic.org/diseases-conditions/depression/basics/definition/con-20032977 (Accessed 5/29/2017).

7. Ibid

8. Merriam-webster.com/dictionary/introspection (Accessed 6/1/2017).

9. http://lungcancer.about.com/od/livingwithlungcancer/tp/Improving-Lung-Cancer-Survival.htm (Accessed 6/1/2017).

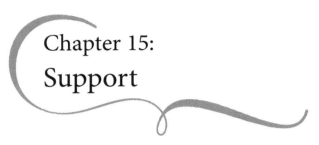

Chapter 15:
Support

Cancer is not always pink. Lung cancer is the number one cancer killer of women.[1]

The general term support is usually divided into the subcategories of physical, financial, emotional, spiritual, and social support. In all cases they imply the provision of some means of help. Literal support to a physical structure may include another structure that bears all or part of the weight by reinforcing or bracing it.

Providing physical support to a person is somewhat similar in that it includes provision of anything that is physically helpful. Examples might include the provision of food, clothing, lodging, rides to the doctor, or taking care of household chores. Financial support literally implies helping the person by gifting or loaning money or the paying or forgiving of debts. Emotional and social support often go together and the terms are sometimes used interchangeably. This type of support includes the provision of things that are emotionally helpful. Examples include a listening ear, understanding, empathy, companionship and encouragement. Spiritual support includes anything that helps the person pursue religious or spiritually meaningful activities. Examples include rides to a place of worship or other religious activities such as reading the Bible (Torah, Quran, etc.), providing spiritually meaningful music, and so on. It is important to note that the support person must support the patient in the patient's chosen religion or spiritual practices and not his or her own.

In healthcare we often talk about the patient's support system. This generally includes everything which contributes to their sense of physical and emotional support as described above but most commonly refers to the people they can rely on for help. Examples of those within a patient's support system may include spouse, family members or other relatives, friends, neighbors, church members, religious leaders, someone who owes them a favor, and anyone else they feel comfortable calling upon for help.

Persons facing a fatal illness can typically benefit from any or all types of support. In fact, having such support has been found to provide a protective function with all types of health. Furthermore, the presence or absence of such support has been identified as a predictor of both morbidity and mortality.

One article that reviewed the results of nearly 150 studies looked at the effect of social relationships on illness and mortality from a wide range of medical conditions.[2] It appeared that people with stronger social relationships had a fifty percent increased likelihood of survival. Looking at cancer alone, another study that compiled nearly ninety studies found that high levels of perceived social support were linked with a twenty-five percent lower relative risk of death.[3]

Having a support network alone can help, but we also need to learn how to ask and receive. After I was diagnosed with cancer, I had many opportunities to practice receiving gifts and expressing gratitude—not always as simple as it sounds. In the American culture, most of us love to give and receive gifts in various forms, yet we are really not very good at it.

Gift-giving can be a last minute act in which we grab and gift something at the last minute in order to not show up emptyhanded, the concern in this case being more for the giver than the receiver. Sadly in such cases, givers miss the opportunity to thoughtfully consider what the receiver really means to him or her. I've experienced the greatest joy in gift-giving when I was able to identify something I knew they would really appreciate and actually use. Sometimes the gifts were odd and inexpensive and observers may have totally missed the point. But when the receiver "gets it" and fully appreciates it, well it's just the best feeling of all. It also helps the receiver truly receive the gift because they know I put some real thought into it and it wasn't a last-minute grab. And the opposite is true as well. When I am gifted with something I really need or really want but maybe never even told anyone (because it was so silly) I am touched deeply. I know they put thought into making their selection and wanted to choose something that "fit" me. This also is a great feeling. Such gift-giving isn't always easy though, especially when buying for the person who "already has everything" or the person is going to die soon. Careful thought is required. I'd like to pretend that I am an excellent giver and have hit the jackpot every time. But that just wouldn't be true. The few times I did hit the jackpot were awesome, and do motivate me to want to do it again. However most of us need help at this which is why I have included in this chapter a section with suggestions for how you might provide gifts of love and support, even from a distance. And as for learning how to fully receive gifts, some of the best advice I've ever received was this. Take a deep breath and relax as you breathe out. Consider the love and thoughtfulness the giver put into this effort (even if the gift is a dud), look them directly in the eyes, and say something that is true and expresses what you think and feel. Something as simple as, "I truly appreciate your thoughtfulness," is fine. If they hit the jackpot then you can embellish even more, but keep it simple and real. "What a thoughtful gift! I love that you knew how much I enjoy _____ and then picked this out just for me." Remember that your genuine gratitude becomes a gift back to the giver.

It's important to keep in mind that one person can't do it all. Helping a family with cancer takes more than one person. You don't need to do it all. Perhaps you are a great listener. Others might enjoy cleaning. Yet others might love gardening. Some might enjoy providing rides. And still others might like working on your car. If everyone who cares, pitches in and does their thing, then most needs will be addressed.

One study used a scoring system that might predict life expectancy of those with advanced cancer in detail to months, weeks and days. This is especially useful for patients who wish to have an accurate prognosis. While no system is perfect, this one has been found to be more accurate than current predictions based on experience, opinion and optimism. This system, developed by Dr. Paddy Stone at St. George's, University of London was based on a study of 1,018 incurable patients referred to palliative care. It took into account age, gender, ethnicity, diagnosis, and disease extent.

According to the authors, this study is the first to benchmark a prognostic scoring system against current best practice but further validation work is required before recommending the scales to be used in routine clinical practice. It is also worthwhile to remember that receiving palliative and hospice care has been shown to increase both longevity and quality of life. So any good scoring system should take this into account along with other factors known to have similar affects.

Offering and Accepting Support

Most adults in the American culture find it easier to offer support to others than to ask for and accept such support for themselves. I believe this is largely because we place such a high value on independence, personal strength, and autonomy in general. Asking for help may be interpreted by some as a sign of weakness. Therefore, most people are extremely hesitant to ask, even when in dire need.

For example, I recall an event many years ago at my church (of the time) where the women were discussing how challenging it can be to maintain the home, take care of young children, and do all of the many things expected of them. So someone was inspired with a clever idea to help women who struggled with housekeeping. They circulated a sign-up list with two categories. One had the heading "I need help cleaning my house" and the other had the heading "I will help someone else clean her house." It wasn't a bad idea. Ideally there would have been enough signatures in both columns to make it all work. However, nearly everyone signed up in the "I will help someone else" column and there were only one or two signatures in the other one. Needless to say, the idea fell flat and was never put into action. I tell the story because it so clearly points out how most Americans are. When it comes right down to it, most of us are much more comfortable offering help to others than asking for help. We may need help. We may be dying of hunger inside a filthy house without a penny to our name, but most of us will do so silently rather than appear weak or needy to others. Asking for help is hard. Humbly accepting help is even harder. Recall my story about being ill with an intestinal virus and reluctantly asking my son and his wife to help change the sheets on my bed. It was not easy to do but in the long run we all benefited by it.

Asking for help can be especially hard for people who have spent years living alone or as single parents. They've grown accustomed to going it alone and have always managed to "make do" and get by on their own. Asking other people for help may feel humiliating and they may fear their request is an imposition. If the person does ask for help, they are likely to only feel okay asking family members, very close friends and persons who owe them a favor.

Being willing to ask for help, for most of us, takes a certain amount of humility and a willingness to appear weak to others, which is never an easy thing. Yet, in practice, the very opposite is often true. To be willing to make oneself appear vulnerable enough to ask for help actually takes a great deal of strength. And then to accept the help that is offered requires another measure of humility. I learned both from experience. Many people would rather suffer alone than to ask for help. I would have. But with experience I realized that it was more hurtful to my loved ones to learn after the fact, that I had needed help and didn't ask. They felt much worse knowing that my needs went unmet. They also felt robbed of the opportunity to have provided something useful. When a person is diagnosed with cancer, especially terminal cancer, other people often want to do something to help but either don't know what to do or are not allowed. In reality when the patient is willing to humble him or herself and fully receive the offered help, even in small things, it becomes a gift to the giver.[3]

Loved ones and friends need to know they have provided something of value. Feeling helpless is one of the things they complain about the most. For this reason, I am dedicating a part of this chapter to providing examples of things one might do to provide support.

Tangible Help

At one time or another we've all heard someone say, or may have said ourselves, "Let me know if you need anything." The person to whom we are speaking always smiles and nods their head, indicating that they will. Yet they almost never do. Why is this? They may worry the person didn't really mean it or that it will pose too much of an imposition. Or perhaps they are simply too embarrassed to ask. Consequently, they don't ask and are left alone with unmet needs.

After undergoing radiation therapy followed by a hellish round of intravenous chemotherapy I found myself in this position. I lived alone in an older house and there were many things that needed to be done. I didn't have the physical energy to do any of them but I could not bring myself to ask for help. My mother did what she could to keep me company and to feed me but she was quite elderly and hesitant to overstep boundaries. My daughter, bless her heart, came by regularly to clean house, feed me, wash the laundry, and do whatever else she could. However, she worked full time, was newly pregnant, had her own home and yard to keep up, plus she tried to accompany me to every appointment. Her two siblings lived far away and this left her shouldering the physical and emotional burden alone. It was just too much and wasn't fair to her, though she would never complain. The day this really hit me, my mother and daughter had come over. Nicole was asking what I had eaten over the past several days while she was working. I reluctantly confessed that I'd survived on chocolate Ensure (a liquid nutritional beverage) and cold cereal. It bothered her much more than it bothered me. But I could see in her eyes how badly she felt. Yet she could only do so much and was not able to stay with me twenty-four hours a day, seven days a week. Knowing how hard she works to hide her feelings I suddenly realized she had been emotionally bearing the entire burden of my illness and all of my needs on her small shoulders. I grasped her hands, looked her in the eyes and said, "It's just too much isn't it?" She immediately teared up but was trying hard not to cry. I embraced her and said, "You've been trying to do it all on your own haven't you?" She nodded as the tears ran down her face. I continued, "You're working full time. You clean my house and then go home to clean your own house. You go with me to every medical appointment. You bring me food. You try to take care of yourself and your baby too. You worry about me and you never complain about how hard this all is. And your brothers live far away, so you feel like it's all on you." She didn't speak but nodded again as the tears flowed. Then I just held her and cried with her for a time. When I spoke I reminded her how much I love and appreciate her and acknowledged that this was all too much for one person to bear. I finally realized that my reluctance to ask for or accept help from others had been selfish and my sweet daughter and my mother were paying the price. I was suddenly motivated to seek help from others and promised her I would do so. I was finally willing to do for her sake what I hadn't been willing to do for my own.

As I began to understand the unfair burden being shouldered by them, I realized I needed to swallow my pride and ask for help. Further, I came to understand how badly my daughter and mother felt when they learned that I wasn't eating properly or had other needs going unmet. Also I realized that I would feel the same way if our positions were reversed and I needed to humble myself and ask for help, for all of our sakes.

The Art of Being With

Many years ago as a nursing student, I had the privilege of attending a small gathering in which our hospital Chaplain spoke about how he had learned the art of being with patients. What I recall from his talk along with what I have learned on my own has served me, and my patients well.

The Art of Being With refers to the physical presence, comfort, reassurance, support, and encouragement one can provide from the simple act of being fully present with them. During this time, you are there one hundred percent for them, for whatever they need. This may include doing things for them if that's what they need. But often all they need is simple companionship. Keep in the back of your mind the needs of nearly everyone to be heard, accepted, validated and responded to. As a personal advocate you can help them, if they desire, to make contact with others to communicate needs with caregivers, family, or friends. While they are verbal or able to communicate in some manner, you can provide a listening ear if they feel like talking. Be an attentive, active listener but do not monopolize the conversation. If they feel like talking, a critical question you can ask is, "What are you hoping for?" This enables you to learn about their needs and wishes for their remaining life. If appropriate, you might communicate with other loved ones and collaborate on a plan for helping the patient achieve their hopes. You may also notice that a common answer is, "I don't know," when you ask what they want or need. Next time try this response: "But if you did know, what would it be?" Yes, I know it sounds silly but it actually works fairly well if you continue to respond in this manner. It forces them to think about it until they do know. At the same time you need to be sensitive. If they really can't think of anything, you can tell them to give it some thought and that you might ask again later.

In many cases, especially as the patient's health rapidly declines, you are simply there as a comforting presence. This may sound too simple. Yet for some of you it might feel too difficult. If you can't be doing or talking or taking some form of action, some of you may become uncomfortable. So to do this properly you must first know yourself and determine if you have the ability to do this. The last thing the patient needs is a nervous, fidgety, restless, uncomfortable person in their room. This is not helpful and can make things worse.

The person who excels at the Art of Being With is someone who is very comfortable in their own skin, who feels at peace and is completely relaxed in the presence of the patient. This person is other-focused, meaning their awareness is on the other person and not themselves. This visitor should let the patient know from the outset what their purpose is. They should invite the patient to do whatever is comfortable (talk, sleep, listen to music, read, or whatever) but do not hover or exert any pressure on them.

To be successful in this process you must have, or be able to establish, a comfortable relationship of trust and rapport. Patients are sometimes able to naturally extend a certain amount of trust to people in certain positions, such as chaplains, clergy and nurses. This is less likely if they don't already have some type of established relationship. If you are already acquainted with the patient in some manner then you can build on this relationship, but take care that you don't revert to making it a gossip session about friends or relatives. After a short time, you will know if it is working. If you are unsure, feel free to ask them if they would like you to return. If they have a reason (of any kind) for why they don't, then graciously wish them well and leave. Don't return (at least in that capacity) and don't take it personally. If the patient is nonverbal and gives you no clues, then perhaps you can inquire with the caregiver, nurse, or family member. Nobody knows for sure what their needs will be when they die. Remember that it is all about them and not about you. If it doesn't work out this time perhaps you can volunteer your time and services in another capacity or with someone else.

Acts of Support

I've been collecting examples of the types of things one might do to support an ill loved one. Listed below are things that others have done for me at various times. The tasks were needed and appreciated. But even more so was the thought and intent behind them. Some were completed by a single person and others required an entire team. In doing things like cleaning my house or bringing food, what people were really saying was that they care about me, were thinking of me, and desired to help in some way. We've all heard the old saying, "It's the thought that counts." Well guess what? It's true. And yet the thought alone conveys nothing unless it's acted upon and communicated in some way.

- Completing minor home repairs.

- Cleaning up my flower beds.

- Coordinating and carrying out a plan to paint my house.

- Scheduling food delivery.

- Cleaning all or part of my house.

- Cleaning out my refrigerator.

- Running errands.

- Picking up groceries.

- Car maintenance including vacuuming the inside and washing the outside, getting snow tires put on or taken off, changing the oil and filter, and getting new windshield wipers.

- Accompanying me to one of my many clinic visits.

- Calling now and then to check in and see how I'm feeling and what I need.

- Dropping more Ensure (or other favorites) by for me to drink.

- Walking my dog.

- Coming by for visits.

- Doing fun things with me like watching a movie, eating, doing crafts, working on a puzzle, etc.

- Supporting my family members knowing they need support as much as I do.

- Making an effort to connect with my children and nurture those relationships; knowing that supporting them is supporting me.

Providing Support from a Distance

A question that has repeatedly arisen is, "How can one provide support from a distance?" In today's mobile world most of us have friends and family scattered all over the country, or even all over the world. It can feel more challenging to respond in helpful ways for such persons in our lives. But I've learned that distance need not be a barrier to providing support although it may change the type of support one provides. Granted, one cannot run local errands, attend medical appointments, or hand-deliver a hot cooked meal when living a thousand miles away. But helpful and meaningful support are still possible. Examples include:

Gifting small inspirational items such as an engraved piece of jewelry, small piece of artwork, or musical CD

Tip: Most effective if you know their taste in jewelry, art, and music.

Personal story: My dear friends at F.A. Davis, publisher of my first three books, sent a card signed by everyone, a beautiful silver, personally engraved bracelet, and an inspirational poem. I loved the thought and the effort and think of them every time I wear the bracelet.

Phone calls

Tip: Time your calls for waking hours, keep calls short so as not to be exhausting.

Personal story: I've enjoyed many calls but one that really stands out is a friend from my early life whom I'd lost contact with. Other close friends and family knew that I had been unsuccessful in locating her so they made the effort to track her down, update her on my health issues, and give her my phone number. This gave her the chance to call me "out of the blue" and surprise me in a very good way.

Phone cards

Tip: Especially nice for someone on a tight budget. Select telephone plans you know will work with their provider and include simple, easy to follow instructions.

Personal Story: I recall, on several occasions, some of my hospital patients whom had been gifted phone cards to make long-distance calls from their room. Not all patients own or have possession of their own cell phones and many are grateful for the means to place calls without worrying about billing issues.

Cards

Tip: Select cards that are inspirational or fit with the patient's religious beliefs or type of humor. If low-tech isn't your thing you can send e-cards of all types through American Greetings and other online sources.

Personal story: I received cards from a friend and coworker every week or two for nearly a year after my diagnosis. They always gave me an emotional boost and let me know that she hadn't forgotten me.

Handmade quilts

Tip: Small quilts work well for naps or snuggling on the sofa; having loved ones sign the quilt makes it especially personal.

Personal story: I received two handmade quilts. One from a former student and her mother (both quilters) made exclusively of nurse-themed fabric (difficult to find!), with a darling handwritten "prescription" label, the other with handwritten notes and signatures from faculty and staff at the college where I'd worked.

Hats and scarves

Tip: Hats are especially nice if the patient has lost their hair from treatment but be sure to check for personal taste and obtain their hat size so they can actually wear it.

Personal story: I've been given several hats. I love the color and style (and thought) but some are too large and others are too small.

Gift cards

Tip: Check with family or close friends to determine patient's taste, physical ability, and preferences. Avoid credit gift cards that deduct a monthly fee. Possibilities are numerous and include grocery stores; restaurants or delis for eat in or take out; spas for a relaxing facial, pedicure, massage, etc.; movie theater; and online sites such as Amazon or various music sites for home shopping.

Personal story: A friend once gave me a credit-type card to shop for whatever I wanted. However, I misplaced it, then eventually found it several months later. When I attempted to use it I learned that nearly all the value was gone because of monthly fees.

Books or magazines

Tip: Check with family to determine the patient's taste and whether something inspirational versus something fun and "escapist" are most appropriate. Send one book or magazine or sign them up for a gift subscription. Also consider audiobooks for people with poor vision.

Personal Story: A friend who has no personal interest in quilting gifted me with a quilting magazine because she heard that I loved quilting. I loved that she selected it based on what she had learned about my interests rather than her own.

E-mails or Twitter

Tip: Easy way to check in, share updates from your life, and let them know you are thinking about them. Consider attachments like personal photos and fun or inspirational cards. Check to make sure patient has computer access, a Twitter account, and skills sufficient to open and read your communication (or has someone there to assist).

Personal Story: I've received numerous e-mails from friends and family since my diagnosis. Those who know me know that I check my e-mail every day and I always feel an emotional boost when I hear from a loved one.

Letters

Tip: Old fashioned, handwritten (or typed) letters are often perceived as more personal than electronic messages, especially with members of the older generation. Check to make sure their eyesight is adequate for reading or there is someone available to assist.

Personal Story: My mother, who has always been a letter writer, lives nearby so I see her fairly often. But when she travels to other parts of the country she usually sends me a brief handwritten letter or card just to let me know she's thinking of me. Regardless of how old I get I always look forward to these long-distant "hugs" from my mama.

Delivery of flowers, plants, fruit basket, etc

Tip: Check for personal preference and potential allergies. For edible items also check for dietary restrictions and potential medication interactions.

Personal Story: Those who know me well know I am sensitive to some fumes and fragrances. Therefore, in lieu of flowers, my preference is for edible arrangements, gourmet coffees and teas, or plants for my garden.

Travel and Visitation

In person visitation may be the perfect gift, but only for a limited number and for close relatives and friends. In some cases, you may be able to help fulfill the last wishes of someone too ill to travel who deeply wish to see a loved one again before they die. You may even be that loved one. Or perhaps you can help the loved one with travel and hotel expenses.

Tips: Do not plan on staying in the ill person's home and do not expect the ill person or their family to host, feed or entertain you. They may already be feeling overwhelmed and exhausted providing for their own needs. Only stay with them if it is clear that this is their preference, you have done so in the past, have a very close relationship, are going to be a caretaker, and there is sufficient room. Contribute to housework, cooking, and other chores. Do not overstay your welcome. Be sensitive to the ill person's physical limitations and needs for quiet and rest. Do not expect them to look, act or feel like they used to. Illness and treatment can have a huge impact on the ill person's appearance, energy level, food tastes, appetite, and mood. Allow them to feel however they feel without imposing your expectations on them. Establish an agreement with them that they will withdraw to their own room to rest whenever they feel the need regardless of whatever else is going on. Be sensitive to the needs of the ill person's children, spouse, and other close family. They may be hurting too and could benefit from your support.

Personal Story: I've always had a very close relationship with my sister. If she comes alone, I prefer to have her stay with me if possible. Having her near is comforting and I am able to relax and be myself with her. Also because of the design of our house, the noise from the living area doesn't conduct (much) to my bedroom. I keep (and use) ear plugs at my bedside and have an agreement with my loved ones that I will retire to my bedroom at any time to rest if I need to. An open bedroom door means they are welcome to join me. A closed door means I am sleeping. If my sister has come with her entire family, which includes grown kids and grandkids, different living arrangements may be preferable.

An Image of Support

It's not always easy to describe to others what I look for in support. An image recently came to me that I want to share because it might help some understand. It occurred to me that I really have no choice about whether or not I take this journey. But I do have some choice in how I take it. As I picture myself walking along I think it would be so great if my family and friends could bring themselves to simply walk along beside me. Some are already doing so. Others are trying. A few are struggling. All I want and need is for them to simply keep me company until it's time for me to cross a bridge that they cannot (yet) cross. In the meantime, let's love each other, cry when we need to, and laugh when we can.

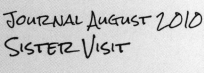

JOURNAL AUGUST 2010
SISTER VISIT

My sister was here for two weeks. It was, and always is, so comforting to have her near. We've always been close though we live far apart. We shared many special moments and used up lots of tissues as we cried together. But we also laughed together as we remembered old times and made bad cancer jokes. We've always shared a wacky sense of humor in our family. It helps us celebrate the good times and cope with the hard times. An important prayer was answered for me during Stephenie's visit. I had asked God to help her and my three kids bond more closely. I hate to think that I might not be here one day but I know it's likely to happen. And it comforts me to know they will have her as a sort of surrogate mom when they have need. I saw this process begin to occur while she was here and I'm confident it will continue.

Journal October 2010 Brother Visit

My younger brother from Texas was here recently. I wish I could see him more but I am grateful that he could come at all. He is an amazing person and during our childhood years, was the brother I spent the most time with. We were sometimes left out of our older siblings' activities because we were "too little." So we frequently played together, usually in the dirt with his cars and trucks, while our older sister and brothers did "big kid" things. We seldom play in the dirt anymore but we still enjoy some great conversations. He always has an interesting perspective on things and a dry, fun sense of humor. He is also incredibly creative in an artsy and techy sort of way; his first love is creating metal sculpted pieces that reflect his unique view of art fused with technology. His creations are interesting and beautiful, and often reflect his unique way of looking at the world.

On this particular visit he gifted me with Petite Fleur (named for the French word for little flower and after a song by Deuter), one of the metal sculptures in his "Dancer" series. I call her Flo. She is beautiful and I love her. She has a place of honor near my fireplace and I think fondly of my brother whenever I look at her.

Hurting Together

Most of the time I think I'm handling things pretty well and yet I notice that I cry easily, often when I don't want to. So maybe I'm not handling things as well as I thought. But I've noticed that the tears typically come when the subject of my family is mentioned. I feel so bad for them and they feel so bad for me and then I feel bad that they feel bad and vice versa. Maybe I make it harder on them by being this way. I surely don't want to. I just don't know how to not feel this way. I think we all just hurt for each other and maybe there is no way around that. I suppose that is part of love; sharing each other's pain. We want to spare each other pain but feel yet more pain when we realize that we cannot. So then we just hurt together and hang on to each other and keep moving forward because what else can we do? But maybe that is how emotional support works.

On this journey we seek to gain maximum value from the time we have. Purely joyful moments of shared humor, laughing at silly things and happy memories. Doing fun, lighthearted things like going to funny movies, playing games, drinking wine, and working on jig saw puzzles, enjoying the now together and wishing with all our hearts that we could stop the clock, at least for a while.

Instead we dive into the moment, gaze into each other in the eyes and say what's on our hearts. We live fully in the now while enjoying rich moments together and create treasured memories for later. It's such an amazingly, agonizingly sweet, painful time. It's wonderful. It's excruciating. It's so very hard and yet I wouldn't trade it for anything. These amazing moments of now are the essence of love. The essence of life. The price is great. The rewards are greater.

Those willing to make themselves vulnerable and move closer to me during this time are indeed paying a great price—and the worst is yet to come, we all know. But I think they would also be the first to say that the sweet rewards are so worth the price. And later, rather than feeling regretful about what they wish they would have done, they will, I hope, wrap themselves in these treasured memories and find comfort, peace and eventually, even joy. That is my wish, prayer and hope for them. These moments that I inadequately attempt to describe, are the times when I feel the most supported.

Finding Support in the Writing of Others

In his little book Mr. Wangerin described himself as the "Professional Patient" spending untold hours sitting in waiting rooms, undergoing examinations and consultations. He pointed out that even though one might have cancer in a specific organ, the entire body "takes the shock," and I thought, "That's so true." He described how the cancer has taken over his "outward" life and has "put death central inside" of him. He states that what he has is not curable but his tumor activity has slowed enough that he and his doctors are now playing a "waiting game" to see when it becomes busier again.[4]

I found his honesty so refreshing and many things he said spoke to my heart and helped me to feel, finally, not alone. He said things I feel, I think, or I wonder about. For example, he commented that he had not prayed for his own healing; a thought probably incomprehensible to many.[5] Why would a person of faith not pray for his own healing? But I have felt the same way and have found it near impossible to explain to others. So when I read his words my heart cried out "Yes! He gets it. He gets it because he's been there. Because he is there!" He strikes me as one who is quite spiritual but not especially religious. I've never met him, but I'm pretty sure I like him.

Being in a sort of quiet time (tumor activity–wise) he was reflecting over the previous two years and anticipating his upcoming death. His hope was that his story might "give shape and meaning to the stories of so many others" with terminal illness, or loved ones with same.[6] What he did for me, I hope to do for others.

JANUARY, 2011
SUPPORT THROUGH
RECONNECTION

I feel as though I've gone through life making connections with other people. Many have no real significance but some do. In those relationships I have somehow given those people a piece of myself; a small sliver of my soul, heart or spirit perhaps. As long as they remain in my life I don't lose it. It is still a part of me because they are still a part of my life. They somehow become an extension of me as somehow my life is enlarged. But when that connection is lost I feel as though they take that part of me with them and my life is left feeling slightly incomplete, perhaps just smaller somehow. If the person played a huge role in my life, like a spouse or very close friend, then the hole left is huge and I grieve the loss for quite some time.

In other cases, the loss isn't felt as acutely. I adapt and go on. Yet when the reconnection occurs at a later time I sense the rejoining of our spirits and feel a new sense of completeness that I didn't know I had been missing. I've noticed this a number of times in the past decade as I've reconnected with good friends from my early life. I don't fully understand it but I think it has something to do with the interconnectedness of all humans; a connection that has always been there (before, during, and after our human lives) that we are largely unaware of. I feel it most acutely with those I am close to but I actually think that on a spiritual level it connects all people; even those we don't know or maybe we know but don't like. It explains why I feel this same sort of contented wholeness when I reconcile with someone that I've been at odds with.

A perfect example is Cindi. The role she's played in my past life had been antagonistic at best. So why would I want to reconcile with her? Why would I now wish to call her friend? Yet I do. And something about it feels right and good. On some level our spirits were connected and needed this healing. I look forward to understanding all of this better when I pass to the next life. I hope it is one of many things that will become clearer to me then.

A Gift of Love in the Form of a Letter

During the first seven months or so after my initial diagnosis I noted a phenomenon that was to become one of the sweetest gifts of my life. As word got out about my illness I began to hear from people I had not been in touch with for a very long time. Phone calls, letters, and e-mails began rolling in. The general purpose for all of them was the same. People who had been a significant part of my life, at some point in my life, began contacting me to tell me about how I had touched them and about the impact of my life upon theirs. What a beautiful thing it was. I heard from friends I'd lost touch with, former high school classmates, and even a former pen pal. These were not the usual newsy letters meant to catch up on recent family and social activities although they might have touched on this. The purpose of these letters and calls was to tell me about how I had impacted their lives, about what I meant to them, and to let me know they were thinking of and praying for me.

It struck me; what an amazing gift, to have friends share from their hearts about how I've touched their lives and what our relationship has meant to them. And I realized that the gift was for both of us. Such a blessing for me but I think it must also be one for them as well. Too often in life we are all so busy working and doing things that we lose track of what is most important. When people take time to write these notes or make these calls they are also pausing to consider what has been most important in their own lives. Along with this they are extending their hearts to me. And if they can do this for me then perhaps they will do the same for other people in their lives. There is something special, nearly magical, that happens when one person opens their heart and extends themselves to another in this way. It is one of the sweetest gifts that one person can give to another. I've had the honor of experiencing this more in my life lately and it helps me to feel God's presence in a profound way.

Chapter 15 Notes

1. Cancer is not always pink. Lung cancer is the #1 cancer killer of women. http://lungcancer.about.com/od/livingwithlung-cancer/tp/Improving-Lung-Cancer-Survival.htm (Accessed 6/4/2017).

2. Petra Rattui. Medical News Today, Cancer / Oncology, Palliative Care / Hospice Care. *Life Expectancy Of Cancer Patients Can Be Predicted Using New Scoring System.* August 25, 2011.

3. https://www.verywell.com/tips-for-improving-lung-cancer-survival-2249249 (Accessed 6/15/2017).

4. Based on the following quote by Stephen Donaldson. "In accepting the gift you honor the giver."

5. Wangerin Jr., Walter. *Letters from the Land of Cancer.* Zondervan. p.9.

6. Wangerin Jr., Walter. *Letters from the Land of Cancer.* Zondervan. p. 102.

   Wangerin Jr., Walter. *Letters from the Land of Cancer.* Zondervan. p. 104

7. Wangerin Jr., Walter. *Letters from the Land of Cancer.* Zondervan. p.11.

8. https://www.verywell.com/tips-for-improving-lung-cancer-survival-2249249 (accessed 2/3/2017).

Chapter 16:
Nonsupport

When I meet people who say—which they do all of the time—
"I must just tell you, my great aunt had cancer of the elbow,
and the doctors gave her ten seconds to live, but last I heard
she was climbing Mt. Everest" and so forth, I switch off early.[1]

We have all bumbled around and said or done the wrong thing with good intentions at some point in our lives. My goal is to bring some of these potential blunders to your awareness so that in the future you might avoid some awkward situations. I will also suggest some alternate words or actions you might substitute. In doing so, I hope to support you in being the supportive person you wish to be to your loved one.

Cancer frightens people and terminal cancer really frightens them. I believe this is because it indirectly reminds them of their own mortality. When a person is diagnosed with an incurable form of cancer, people typically want to say something caring and supportive. But the fatal nature of the illness often becomes a stumbling block for them, making conversation feel awkward. In an effort to ease the tension and make everyone feel better, they sometimes speak without thinking which can backfire.

You can probably remember at least once in your life being the speaker or the listener in such a situation. Something is said and it quickly becomes apparent that the speaker has "put his foot in his mouth." An awkward silence often follows, but at other times the speaker goes merrily on their way without a clue they have just embarrassed, insulted, or hurt someone. Generally, people will shrug it off knowing that the speaker meant well. Often the things they say are what have become known as clichés or platitudes; flat, shallow, dull, or trite, overused remarks that are meant to help, but don't.

Clichés and Platitudes

Wangerin noticed even before he began chemotherapy; people issuing oft-heard, well-meant but shallow and overused clichés and platitudes when they didn't know what else to say. He noticed it caused him to feel an increased distance between them and himself, which was probably the opposite of what was intended.[2]

I can relate to this. I know that people usually mean well. But it still gets tiresome, especially when my energy is low. And Wangerin is correct. It does create a feeling of more, rather than less, distance. Sometimes when such things are said I notice various thoughts running through my mind that are probably best left unsaid and are not what the speaker meant for me to think. Some examples follow:

Comments that seem to trivialize the situation rather than acknowledging its significance or potential severity:
    "I'm sure you'll be fine."
    "They are discovering new cures every day."
    "You will probably outlive the rest of us."
    My thoughts: I'm thinking that you probably don't understand

the severity of the situation or the significance of what I'm going through.

Telling people what they must do:
"You have to keep fighting."
"You must not give up."
"You need to go to XYZ clinic."
My thoughts: I already feel overwhelmed. I feel pressured by family, friends and myself. I don't need one more person telling me what I must do. Also, a time may come when I do not have the strength or desire to fight anymore. Please don't make me feel like a failure when that time comes. There is a time for most people when giving up, more accurately called acceptance, is the right thing to do. At this point the most loving thing you can do is accept and support my choice.

Offering unsolicited medical advice:
"Make sure you find the right doctor (or other health practitioner)."
"You should go to ____ (big city and/or famous cancer treatment facility)."
"Don't trust mainstream medicine. Doctors don't want you to get well or they'd be out of business."
"You need to take _____. (juices, tonics, herbal supplements, "natural" medicines, special vitamins, filtered water and the like)."
"Cancer cannot live in a high alkaline environment so you need to change your body's pH."
"You can cure cancer with a special diet (vegetarian, vegan, dairy-free, asparagus, whole food, anti-oxidant, organic, "natural," etc.)."
My thoughts: I cannot try everything on the market and it wouldn't be good for my body if I did. Many such treatments are not approved, may be unsafe, and may interact with my current medication or treatment. I have discussed my options with my

healthcare providers and we've come up with a plan that I feel good about.

Please don't make assumptions about my situation which may be more complex than you realize and don't give medical advice unless you are a physician (and have been asked). It is rude and disrespectful to make derogatory comments about physicians in general and my physician in particular. I've already gathered data, analyzed options, and agonized about what to do. I will work with my own healthcare provider to establish the treatment plan I feel is best.

Such comments imply I have given little thought to the situation and feel disrespectful of my intelligence and my choices. Please remember that a healthcare provider or medical facility is not better just because of its location (in the big city or another country). If I agree to go elsewhere for care are you going to pay for my travel expenses (air fare, gasoline, hotel stay, and food)? Are you going to house sit for me, look after my pets, collect my mail, pay my bills, keep up my yard, and reimburse me for lost work time?

Various comments regarding the importance of attitude:
"Just keep thinking positive."
"Remember, mind over matter."
"Keep your chin up."
My thoughts: This over-simplifies a complex situation and implies that I may have a poor attitude. Furthermore, it seems to suggest that it's my own fault if I die from cancer (for having a poor attitude). People die every day from countless causes. Did they all fail to think positively enough? I recognize there is power in a positive attitude, but this is not always easy to do. I need to be able to feel how I feel at any given time without being criticized for having a bad day, or for simply being realistic.

Comments implying that it is simply a matter of having enough faith, attending the right church or praying the right way:

"God will heal you if you have enough faith."

"You should come to church with me so our elders can lay hands on you and pray for healing."

My thoughts: Not everyone is equally confident or comfortable "claiming" that God will heal them. This may or may not have anything to do with their amount of faith. They may hear God telling them something else. They may be seeking God's will but may not yet be clear what it is. Perhaps they know but aren't comfortable talking about it. Or perhaps they don't believe in God at all. In any case you can support them through silent prayer, and by respecting their beliefs and their privacy.

An insight that occurred to me very early on was that it takes a whole different level of faith and confidence to believe (and claim) God will heal me, than to make similar claims for someone else. Because this time it's me. It's my body. I have much more personally at stake than when it's someone else. To claim something I don't feel sure of feels false. I'm not at a place in my life where I can play games with God.

Comments that imply people bring cancer on themselves and/or fail to be healed as a result of their own failures (bad habits, sin, bad karma, stupidity, ignorance):

"This must be God's will."

"Oh, how long did you smoke?"

"Your body will heal itself if you just give it what it needs."

"You need to get right with God."

"He brought this on himself you know (spoken to someone else)."

My thoughts: Persons who make these types of comments probably mean well and are trying to be supportive. But it's important to know that such comments can sometimes feel pushy, intrusive, or insulting to the person with cancer. Do you believe all of your or your loved one's illnesses are brought on by sin or lack of faith? Every time one of your loved ones died, did they bring it on themselves? Upon hearing such comments, persons with cancer may feel there is an unspoken implication that if they are not healed it's because of their failure to perform the suggested actions.

Comments to not give up for whatever reason:

"Don't give up! They produce new cures every day, and yours might be right around the corner."

"You can't die! Your family needs you."

My thoughts: The first comment might well be true, but statistically the odds are extremely unlikely. Medical science is continually making progress. But getting new drugs and treatments through the research and development phase and eventually approved for use is a very S-L-O-W process. Furthermore, there are hundreds of types of cancer and what treats one doesn't necessarily treat another.

Also, though we don't like to admit it, people die every day. I don't want to leave my family, but it may be out of my hands. Please don't make me feel worse about it than I already do.

After reading the section above, if you still don't know what to say, try a sincere, "I'm so sorry you are going through this," and leave it at that.

What if you are the patient? What should you say in response when other people make silly or annoying comments?

The following suggested responses are for the ill person to use if they seem appropriate but only when the person involved doesn't take subtle hints. Take a deep breath and remember that most people mean well. If they are too pushy consider giving them a gentle dose of the truth. It may help them think before they speak up the next time. Some possible responses include:

"I realize you are trying to cheer me up, but it just doesn't feel that simple to me."

"I'm sure you mean well. Thanks for wanting to encourage me."

"My cancer is very different from (person's name). But thanks for trying to cheer me up."

"I do try to keep a positive attitude, but it isn't always an easy thing to do. What I really need are people who love and support me regardless how I'm feeling."

"I'm struggling to face my mortality while maintaining my faith. It's not always an easy thing."

"I appreciate your concern and/or your prayers."

"Making treatment decisions in the face of a potentially fatal illness is more challenging than most people can imagine and is not something I do lightly."

"I appreciate your care and concern."

"I hope you can appreciate my need for privacy regarding my personal healthcare choices."

"If we are going to be totally honest for a moment let's admit that neither of us knows for sure what God's will is. However, I appreciate your prayers on the matter."

"In most cases nobody knows for sure what causes cancer."

"Of course smoking is a bad idea. We all know that; but nobody deserves to go through this whether they've smoked or not."

"We don't like to admit it, but sooner or later everyone dies. How else are we supposed to get to heaven?"

"If perfect faith and the perfect diet will make us live forever then how are we to get to heaven?"

"Do you really think a doctor or clinic is better just because they are located in the big city?"

"Your attitude toward doctors and the medical profession is pretty sad. I happen to trust and respect my doctor."

"Thanks for your concern. I've done my homework and I'm comfortable with my choices for medical care."

"My physician and I are in agreement about what I should and shouldn't put into my body."

"I'm not comfortable with mega-doses of vitamins and supplements because they can interfere with other medications, and can sometimes cause more harm than good."

"Our kidneys work hard to keep the acid/base balance in our bodies right where it needs to be. Taking large doses of alkaline substances (like baking soda) can be quite dangerous."

If none of these responses suits you, consider giving them a brief smile and change the subject. They should get the message.

Religious Nonsupport

Sometimes, under the guise of support, religious individuals will share their beliefs with ill persons. The intention may be to provide a gesture of care and concern. But tread carefully. This is sacred ground and such gestures should never be forced on a nonconsenting individual. Sadly, the more vulnerable the person, the more likely some are to offer such support. I've personally known of people who visited the elderly in long-term care facilities or even hospitals with the goal of coercing them into "deathbed conversions." This practice is considered unethical and is generally not allowed unless the patient has invited the visitors. Faith is a very personal thing. Efforts to impose one's faith on patients or member of any vulnerable population are not appropriate and are rarely appreciated. Furthermore, people who want such visits will generally have already made arrangements to meet with the clergy or members of their own faith.

Remember that you may pray silently and privately for anyone you wish. God hears all prayers whether spoken verbally or silently.

People who insist on making an uninvited public display of prayers or other religious activities may be more concerned about their own agenda than the well-being of the patient.

JOURNAL MAY 2010
THINKING POSITIVE?

My dear friend Mollie is determined to cure me with her filtered water and nutritional supplements. I appreciate her intent. I know she cares and is trying to support me in the best way she knows . . . but it is not the way that I need. It is so frustrating when she tries to "educate" me with tidbits of medical information, usually taken out of context and provided by her water filter company; which surely has its own agenda. It feels weirdly ironic that she instructs me to "unplug" from my medical knowledge in order to believe what she is selling. Apparently I am not allowed to hope in medicine or science but should place my faith in nutritional supplements? Very little of it makes any sense but she can't see it. It leaves me feeling frustrated in a way I cannot describe and I seem unable to adequately explain it to her. I have no desire to hurt or insult her, yet I feel that is what she has done to me. She has read a few very biased articles promoted by her water filter and herbal supplement companies and is sure I will also be convinced by reading them. Well I did, and I'm not. Meanwhile, she seems to totally discount my years of education and work in healthcare. I am the ignorant one? Is my skepticism a lack of faith? She tells me, "The body knows how to heal itself if we just give it the right support." What I hear is that if I do not recover it will be my fault for not giving my body the right support (as she defines it).

The Alkaline Myth

I've been asked many times about using water filters, or other strategies such as alkaline diets or even ingesting baking soda to prevent or cure cancer. Those who sell the filters and certain supplements will tell you that "cancer cannot survive in an alkaline environment" and therefore their products will protect or save you by raising your pH (making your body more alkaline).

There is no credible evidence that drinking alkaline water has any benefit. And the filtration systems are absurdly expensive. As far as I can tell only the people selling them have "evidence" that they work. I've read some of their literature and plenty of other articles from reputable sources that discount them all.

Regardless what we eat or drink our body (especially our kidneys) works very hard to keep our blood pH within the very narrow normal range of 7.35–7.45. Any higher or lower is not good and can make you ill. When people talk about testing their pH (as the water filter people do) what they are testing is saliva pH or in some cases urine pH. Normal urine pH varies between 5.0 and 8.0. Normal pH for saliva averages 7.0 but is variable. The one that matters most is blood pH.

When we are healthy, our blood is already slightly alkaline, just a little higher than the totally neutral pH of 7.0 on the pH scale, which runs 0 to 14. Anything below 7.0 is acidic. Anything higher is alkaline. An example of a totally neutral fluid is distilled water. So by comparison our blood must be slightly alkaline. Fortunately, the kidneys normally do an excellent job of keeping us where we need to be. What you eat or drink has little or no effect on blood pH (as long as you have healthy kidneys). This is actually a good thing because we'd all have killed ourselves long ago if we could change our pH so easily. During some types of illness our blood sometimes becomes mildly acidic but that does not mean raising our blood pH is going to cure us. If the underlying problem is corrected, the body will correct the pH level. Trying to change your body's pH by ingesting large amounts of acidic or alkaline substances is foolish and can be dangerous for people with certain health problems. The safest advice I can offer is, "Don't go there."

Will filtered water or nutritional supplements hurt you? Yes, they will both hurt your budget because they are usually quite expensive. Having said that, I will concede that the water shouldn't hurt you but the supplements could be problematic depending upon what's in them, what medical conditions you have and which medications you are on. To be safe you should always consult with your doctor before taking them.

Journal December 2010
Feeling Abandoned . . .

I hadn't heard from Mollie for many months. She had been a very close friend, or at least I thought so. Now I'm not sure, because she evaporated from my life not long after my diagnosis. I assume it had something to do with my not agreeing to abandon medical (scientific) care and employ her recommended methods instead. These included drinking filtered water and taking handfuls of nutritional supplements. I tried repeatedly to explain my perspective but she never seemed to understand. I could have gotten past the irrational arguments and even the disrespect of my education and my career. The problem was that after saying what a great friend I am, how she wants to keep me in her life, and how much she loves and values me, she proceeded to disappear from my life once it became clear I wasn't going to use her products. Then there's the grand finale. A few months later she reported to a mutual friend that I had "decided to die." How in the world did she draw that conclusion? Accepting death as an inevitable fact of life and "deciding to die" are quite different. I was deeply saddened by her response and her choice to disappear from my life at a time when I most needed her. It still baffles me.

Unsolicited advice and other things that annoy me.

Everyone advises me to "think positive" and keeps reciting their stories about someone they know who was cured and went on to live to a ripe old age. Of course I would like the same to be true for me too. But I suspect it is easier to feel certain of a miraculous outcome for someone else than it is for oneself. At least for me that is the case. I could voice positive beliefs for someone else because if I'm wrong—well it would be unfortunate, but not the end of the world—at least not for me.

But things are different now. We aren't talking about someone else. We are talking about me and my life. There is so much more at stake from my point of view and I just can't bring myself to voice a certain belief in something I feel uncertain about. I hope that doesn't mean I lack faith. I do believe God will see me through this—but to what end I am not certain.

Looking great

Here's another question to ponder. Why does it bug me when people tell me that I "look great?" I know they mean well. And yes, I suppose it's nicer than if they said I look terrible. But I know it's a new "cancer" thing and I can't help but wonder what's behind it. I try to just say "thank you" and accept it as a compliment or at least as a positive comment. Yet they say it almost as if they are surprised. Like they expected me to immediately start looking terrible from the moment of diagnosis. I'm never sure what to say. I never used to get so many "compliments." And trust me, I really don't look all that great. So having a somewhat warped sense of humor, the responses below often flit though my mind.

"So you think I should immediately start looking bad?"

"What is someone with cancer supposed to look like?"

"Oh, well I will eventually look really awful so please stay tuned."

"Are you doubting the accuracy of my diagnosis?"

"Makeup does wonders. You should have seen me when I got up this morning."

(I've actually used this last one a few times.)

Website disappointment

Because there weren't any support groups in town that met my needs I decided to look online. My first few searches yielded a variety of groups but none came anywhere close to what I wanted. Eventually I found one that seemed promising. It was fairly specific in that it was for people with lung cancer and even had different areas for those with various stages of cancer.

My hope when I first found this website was that I might find others who would be interested in having the sort of conversations that I long to have. Not so much about endless hunts for cures or alternative forms of treatment. But rather, about our thoughts, hopes, and fears related to the possibility of dying, what people think about the afterlife, and how they cope with various challenges. I want to talk with others in a similar place who are realistic about what is happening. I'd love to have discussions about near-death experiences, deathbed visions, and angels. I'd love to talk about what we think our final transition might be like, what we hope comes next and what each person's perception of an afterlife is like. I'd like to talk about coping skills, and how people deal with everyday issues like fatigue, anorexia, or waking during the night feeling alone and frightened. I'd love to discuss how we make the most of each day (aside from trying to "think positive") and boost our own spirits when we feel down.

After spending some time on the website, I found myself with mixed feelings about it. It felt useful to connect with others traveling a similar path, to share thoughts and stories. It was especially nice to compare experiences with other Tarceva users. However, because I'm not just a patient but also a nurse and an educator, I sometimes feel compelled to share information when others ask questions, or worse yet, spread incorrect and possibly dangerous information. I want them to understand how things work and why I think a certain course of action is wise or not, but that can be an exhausting process, because I'm not usually one to give a quick, simple answer, and already I find myself growing weary.

It also becomes rather repetitive since one who joins the website this week wasn't around for the in-depth discussion of the same subject last week. It's nobody's fault but is just the way it works. People are often frightened and worried and who can blame them? I was worried and frightened in the beginning too. And though I had a career as a fixer (nurse), I do not have the time and energy to try to fix everyone there. And, more to the point, I cannot fix them. Most of them have a terminal prognosis, as do I. We cannot fix each other. That shouldn't be the purpose of the group, but, based on the various discussions, it seems to be a common expectation.

I also find that I'm spending more and more time defending physicians and the medical profession in general. There is a fair amount of doctor-bashing from people who have had a bad experience. So now they've decided that all doctors are simply out to make a fast buck and don't care about their patients, a perspective I do not agree with. Such negativity is the last thing other members of the group need to hear.

Last of all, I'm not getting my own needs met, which was the reason for my search in the first place. I find that I quickly move into the "educator" role which I suppose is my comfort zone, but is not why I'm there. There seems to be little interest in the subjects I would like to pursue, although I did attempt to start a discussion by asking how they have learned to ask for support. It met with a lukewarm response which is really sad because it's something that everyone struggles with. I concluded that either they haven't figured it out or were uncomfortable discussing it. It seems as if they preferred to focus on the negative while preaching the positive. I don't know if that makes sense but most conversations are quite depressing—talking about complications and side effects, or doctor bashing while chanting their on-going mantras of "don't give up," "doctors are wrong," "anyone can be healed," and so on. Only when someone writes about accepting that the end has come for a loved one (who's now beyond writing him/herself) do the others then (mostly) concede the inevitable and offer prayers for a peaceful death. Yet even in those cases there are always some who continue their chants of "Fight, fight!" and "Don't give up!" or offering continued advice for other forms of treatment. I feel quite frustrated when I read such posts.

JOURNAL JULY 2011
FRUSTRATION

I noticed that people on the website generally disappear after a few years. A rare few improve but only those in the stage I and II discussion groups. Stage III is iffy. Some get better. Most don't. In stage IV where I hung out for a while, nobody recovers. And it's the big white elephant in the room that nobody talks about.

Am I really the only one on this planet that thinks this way? Am I so unusual in accepting my own mortality? Or am I just failing to be politically correct in end of life conversation, even among a crowd of people who are all deemed terminal?

The people I get most annoyed with are the "intruders" on the web site. People whom I believe, have no right to be there. Some guy there to promote his XYZ water filters. He doesn't have cancer. He doesn't have a clue. He just wants to make money off of vulnerable people. Another guy, who I think means well, but is almost as annoying in a different way. He is well read and had researched alternative therapies up the kazoo. Apparently he had some form of cancer many years ago. He is a writer and has written many books (by his own accounts) on the subject of alternative treatments, nutritional supplements and the like. By his report he's been in remission all these years. This may be true, but I can't help but question his motives in being on this site. He's in the stage IV group where the sickest (most vulnerable) people are. He preaches that anyone with any form or stage of cancer can be healed if they simply pursue the health practices he describes. Forgive my cynicism, but might his real agenda just be to sell his books? I mean really, if his cancer was healed so very long ago why would he still feel compelled to spend so much time on this web site? This is generally a place where people with cancer go to give and receive support from one another and not a place where healthy people hang out.

Then there are those who have read a few books or articles (of questionable sources) and are now the experts on everything. Like the gal who keeps trying to "educate" others on the site with her "alkaline mantra." She is an ignorant boob who thinks she knows all and is doing more harm than good there. But she is also incredibly stubborn and not teachable. So it's pointless to carry on debates with her.

Hopefully there are better internet support groups out there now but after my experience I gave up looking. I had entered the site seeking honest conversation from others on similar journeys and it didn't work out. But I still like the idea. I think such a site could work well if the moderators have a clear vision of their purpose and the help they need to make it work. Helpful contributors would include but not necessarily be limited to experts in home care resources such as nurse case managers, and medical experts such as nurses and doctors in oncology, palliative care and hospice care. To promote effective group interaction expert facilitators in virtual group process would be needed. They could help moderate conversation threads, keep people on topic and allow them to vent without trashing an entire profession. They could request expert opinions on topics of discussion when needed and promote the sharing of positive coping strategies. I would have loved finding such a site when I was first looking. I doubt I'm the only one.

Chapter 16 Notes

1. Christopher Hitchens, http://www.brainyquote.com/quotes/ keeywords/cancer_2.html (Accessed 6/5/2017).

2. Wangerin Jr., Walter. *Letters from the Land of Cancer*. Zondervan, 2017. p.32.

Chapter 17:
Final Hope

Last words of Thomas Edison: "It is very beautiful over there."[1]

Last words of Steve Jobs: "Oh wow! Oh wow! Oh wow!"[2]

As Doris began to slip away, she reported seeing things. Dr. Barrett said the young woman looked eagerly towards a part of the room and as she did, a large smile crossed her face. "Oh lovely, lovely," she said. "What is lovely?" asked Dr. Barrett. "What I see," said Doris. "Lovely brightness— wonderful beings."[3]

I've pondered what I might write that would be the most encouraging, comforting and inspirational for anyone who's stuck with me long enough to get to this final chapter. We are each different but the best I know is to share with you what has most encouraged, comforted and inspired me. Obviously a large part of this is my faith, much of which I've already shared. This chapter will focus on other topics of a spiritual nature that have significantly strengthened my belief in the afterlife and significantly decreased my fear and anxiety regarding death and dying.

Some of the things I share may seem a bit farfetched to some of you and you may find yourself responding with skepticism. That's fine. I once had the same response and I still don't necessarily believe everything I read or hear about. All I ask from you is that you proceed with an open mind and see if there is anything here that might be of value to you. If you decide there is not, then you've lost nothing but a few minutes of your time. On the other hand, if there are any pearls here that enrich the remainder of your life in some way, then your time reading and pondering this will have been well worth it. Give it a chance. Your hopes for your future may be bolstered and my hopes in writing this book will have been realized.

There is More

I find it odd that there seems to be such continuing debate among the medical and scientific communities about whether there is life after death given the fact that a majority of Americans (eighty-one percent) believe in an afterlife.[4] Even globally, over half of the world's population are believers.[5]

I have always believed in life after death, but more so now than ever before. Part of what has caused this surge in my belief is the information I will try to convey to you in this chapter. I've always been an avid reader but since my diagnosis, have probably read at least sixty books on various subjects related to life after death and will now try to convey the essence and key points of what I've learned. I will also provide references and a Suggested Reading List at the end of this book for you to do further study if you wish. I hope to pique your interest enough that you will want to explore further for yourself. I certainly had to.

I'm the sort of person who feels compelled to do my own research, especially if the subject is important to me. After I've read many books and other literature written by those with experience, knowledge, or expertise, then I ponder it for a while. Usually I then feel compelled to read the more interesting and more credible sources at least once more, note the trends, and then use my own brain and common sense to decide where I believe the truth lies. I also pray about it and ask God to confirm or clarify whatever issue I'm pondering. This really does seem to help me. I encourage you to follow whatever steps work for you.

Near Death Experiences (NDEs)

An NDE is said to have occurred when a person nearly or actually dies but is later revived. During the death state they have no pulse and no breath for a period of at least five to fifteen minutes (sometimes longer).[6] During the experience they maintain an intense awareness of what is occurring and it remains crystal clear in the person's mind regardless of how much time has since elapsed. The experience has a deep impact on them and they may exhibit significant personality changes including those related to values, beliefs and life focus from that time onward.[7]

Normally when a person is deprived of oxygen for more than five minutes, brain damage occurs. The amazing thing about an NDE is that no matter how long the person was dead they not only experience no brain damage but often return with brain enhancement.[8] Accounts vary widely but precipitating events include motor vehicle accidents, illnesses of all types, or injuries that lead the person to the brink of death.

No two NDEs are exactly alike but an assortment of elements have been identified.[9] It seems to me that we really ought to listen to what these people are saying, since they have information that might well shed some light on what we all want to know. It doesn't mean you or I must believe every story we hear. If you discounted even half of them or more, that still leaves a significant number of accounts that have something important to tell us. I, for one, am inclined to listen.

Most NDEs include only a few of the following elements. The more elements involved, the "deeper" the NDE is said to be.

- Hearing yourself pronounced dead.
  By medical personnel, friends, or bystanders.

- Feelings of peace and quiet.
  The person may or may not continue to hear normal noise but usually experiences a sensation of peacefulness beyond anything he or she has ever experienced before.

- Hearing unusual noises.
  Instead of hearing expected noises or total silence, some people hear buzzing or clicking noises or musical sounds.

- Seeing a dark tunnel.
  Occasionally described as a light tunnel, or a tunnel with bright or colored flashing lights. Some saw other people in it. But more often it was a dark tunnel with a light at the end. They often described a feeling of moving along the tunnel at great speed and felt wind rushing by. The light was described as being brighter than any they had ever seen, yet did not hurt their eyes. They also described the light as conveying pure love, intelligence, and peace, and was the most wonderful thing they had ever experienced.

- Finding yourself outside your body.
  During an out-of-body experience (OBE) the individual feels aware of leaving his or her body and being able to see it from a distance. This is one of the most common experiences.

- Meeting "spiritual beings."
  Sometimes identified as spiritual figures or beings of light they are usually associated with that person's religion and may be referred to as angels, Jesus, Buddha, or Mohammed.

These beings usually communicate love, peace, patience, and acceptance.

- A panoramic life review.
  Descriptions vary but somehow the person's entire life is reviewed so that he or she can see or even relive it. What's more amazing is that they also experience the effect of their actions on other people from those persons' point of view. Some even describe being aware of the ripple effect of their actions as they impact others known to the person they effected. Other beings may be standing by in a supportive and loving manner. The person is judged only by him or herself.

- Sensing a border or limit to where you can go.
  Somehow they know that if they go beyond the border they will be unable to return to life. The border is represented in numerous ways; a river, stream, fence, gate, tree, etc.

- Coming back into your body.
  Often, but not always, through the head. Often described as painful or uncomfortable. Bodily feelings such as pain and temperature extremes immediately return.

- Ineffability, beyond the limits of any language to describe.
  Indescribable.

- Frustrating attempts to tell others what happened.
  Because the experience is ineffable, words cannot adequately describe it. Listeners are often skeptical and may assume the person was hallucinating or confused.

- Subtle "broadening and deepening" of their life afterward.
  The realization that things they valued before are not very important and are now replaced by love and the desire to help others. Many described themselves as suddenly and profoundly changed and believed they would never be the same.

- Elimination of the fear of death.
  Because they now feel sure that death is not the "end" but rather a transition to an even better realm of existence, they lose fears they may have associated with it. Most look forward to returning one day.

- Corroboration of events witnessed while out of body.
  Accurately recounting the actions or statements by medical personnel who previously tried to revive them. Accurately recounting actions and statements of family or friends in other locations from where their body was.

- A realm where all knowledge exists.[10]
  While in "heaven" or a spiritual place they have all questions answered about the meaning of life and such.

- Cities of light.
  Described beautiful cities seen from a distance that emanated a heavenly light.

- A realm of bewildered spirits.
  Some experienced unpleasant scenes with dark, evil beings and harsh voices. Even so, most say it has had a positive impact on their life.

- Supernatural rescues.
  Occasionally people return having been healed from cancerous tumors or other illnesses. Stories of NDEs by drowning sometimes describe a bodiless pair of hands that reached down and pulled them from the water. Other stories describe angelic beings that rescued them from dangerous situations or threatening persons.

Ruth

While I was discussing NDEs one day with a relative, she surprised me with a true story of her own. She described a day when she was just twelve years old and was playing at a lake with her cousins and friends. There were many children splashing in the water while all of the adults watched from the shore. Since she didn't know how to swim, Ruth was always careful to remain in shallow water. But on this day, the algae had grown so thick that it made discerning the water's depth very difficult. Without meaning to she had paddled out too far when another child hit her inner tube causing her to flip into deep water. The next thing she knew she was in water over her head. Before she had time to feel frightened she saw two white arms reaching for her and heard an audible voice saying, "You are going to be ok and I will never leave you." The next thing she knew she was standing in shallow water, facing the beach. Ten years passed before she shared her story with anyone. As she described the events of that day that occurred over fifty years ago, she exclaimed that "it is just as vivid today as the day it happened."

Lasting Transformation

I first met Samantha and her twin when they were infants. Her remarkable story began even earlier when her mother was hospitalized on bed rest and IV medications to prevent preterm labor. This bought them more time to mature. Even so, they were born early at 32 weeks (40 is normal). At one point in the process it became clear that Sam was in trouble. She developed a grade 4 intraventricular bleed (stroke) and her blood pressure dropped to zero. Needless to say, this created an extremely traumatic event for Sam and her family with many tears and prayers to follow. Her twin was fine but doctors feared that Sam would not be. In fact, her prognosis was quite grim and her parents were warned to "prepare themselves for the worst". How does one do that?

In the course of events Sam experienced a NDE that she was unable to tell her parents for several years. One day, after learning to speak, Sam told them about it. She remembered crawling up a beautiful celestial stairway surrounded by angels and other divine beings. Eventually she reached the top where she enjoyed a divine cuddle with Jesus. Afterwards she was returned to her body in perfect health. In the years following she has exhibited many of the signs of one who has undergone a life-changing NDE. Some included being exceptionally bright which allowed her to complete high school and college early. Creative talents include a beautiful singing voice and photography skills. Others include certain psychic skills along with a warm and outgoing personality which sometimes leads perfect strangers to approach her and share personal, spiritual experiences. Over the years it also became apparent that she and her brother shared an unusual bond in which she experiences mental or intellectual aspects of an event while he experiences the physical aspects.

NDE Trends

As you might expect, most people are initially anxious and fearful about the dying process and the knowledge of their impending death. Most have no clear idea what to expect but have heard enough stories throughout their lives to be somewhat apprehensive. Death is something that is easy to joke about when it feels very far away. But when it looms near, jokes and pretense fade away. People become acutely aware that there is no escape and may worry about what is ahead. I have personally heard a number of people comment that they are not especially afraid of death itself, but do have some anxiety about the dying process. I realized this was largely true for me as well. Even once I made peace with the "death" part of the deal, I still had questions and admittedly some fear about the "dying" part. Exactly how will I die? What will it be like? None of us wants to suffer and yet we believe sometimes people do. So we are left feeling vulnerable and out of control.

I would probably be lying if I claimed to have overcome one hundred percent of my fear and anxiety. But most of it has melted away. It's happened slowly as I've learned more and more about other people's near death experiences and pre-death experiences. They are the closest things we have to go on regarding the topics of dying and a possible afterlife, so I decided to pay attention to those who report them. NDEs are much more common than most realize with an estimated eight to fifteen million Americans having undergone an NDE.[11] In the past, people didn't talk about them much. So what may seem to be a recent phenomenon is not really something new. It's just that more people are finally willing to talk about them. Previously most people kept their NDE experience a closely guarded secret because of concern about what others would think and say. Fortunately, the NDE experience is slowly becoming better known and more accepted.

One of the first things I noticed when I read Life After Life approximately fifteen years ago, was that I felt comforted and my fears related to dying and death diminished significantly.[12] My interest had been piqued so I continued reading. I found many interesting things to ponder in all of the NDE accounts, but one of the first big takeaways for me was noting that for the most part, people seemed to be spared the most awful parts of the dying experience. The scary things I had envisioned about dying didn't turn out to be as scary as I had expected. And some things about it were actually intriguing. It made me curious and left me wanting to know more. So I kept finding other books to read.

When I read about Dr. Mary Neal's NDE through drowning

I found it very interesting to note that she didn't describe some horrific experience that was as frightening and physically torturous as I'd always imagined. In Dr. Neal's case, as she realized she was about to drown she reached out to God, asking for His divine intervention. In response she immediately experienced an overwhelming feeling of peace and calm and the sensation of being held and comforted in someone's arms. She continued to feel calm and comfortable as she experienced a life review and eventually felt her soul leave her body, then exit the water where she was greeted by a group of other souls and the most intense joy she had ever experienced.[13] I noticed the same trend in accounts where people suffered other forms of traumatic death. So often they simply found themselves out of their bodies, watching from a distance. Those involved in motor vehicle accidents might remember a loud crashing sound or flashing headlights and then their next awareness was of being outside of the car looking on. This allowed them to skip much of the misery I always feared they suffered.

Another common trend I noticed is that there wasn't necessarily a clear point in the story where it was obvious to the person that he or she had died; at least not in the way I'd always envisioned. Their "conscious" thoughts and observations continued on in an unbroken manner and it often didn't even dawn on them that they had died until sometime after the fact. Typically, this realization came when they found themselves looking downward at their own body or noticed that others could not see or hear them. In nearly every case, this experience was followed by travel through a tunnel or alongside a spiritual being of light to a place where they were greeted by previously deceased loved ones. In some cases, a loved one was the first being they encountered and that person escorted them on their journey. The accounts are all similar yet each is unique in some way.

As I began learning about NDEs I found them comforting in

the sense that the information lessened my grief regarding loved ones I've lost. One of the things that had always haunted me was imagining how they must have suffered. Now I find I am less bothered by this thought as I now believe that God intervened to spare them from much of it. And the thought hits me; why wouldn't He? I know I would do whatever I could to spare my own children from suffering. So why wouldn't God do the same for us? We are his children. It also comforts me to consider that He may do the same for me when it's my turn.

A Missed Opportunity

If I hadn't seen this one myself, I probably wouldn't have believed it. At least not at the time. I might believe it now, depending on who was telling me.

I had been working regular twelve-hour nights on the medical-oncology unit of our local hospital for about a year when I was assigned to care for Joe, a fifty-six-year-old man diagnosed with renal (kidney) cancer. He had been hospitalized for pain control and was expected to die soon. When I assessed him near the beginning of my shift he was awake, oriented, and verbal. He stated his pain was currently well controlled since he was taking an extended-release form of oral morphine and his only complaint at the time was of the severe fatigue that never left him. I helped him settle in for the night and then left him to rest as I checked on my other patients. I checked on him approximately ninety minutes later and he was sleeping with calm, regular breathing. So I left to tend to other patients. Near midnight I stepped quietly into his room to check on him again and noted he wasn't breathing. His status was "no code" which means he had made the request to not have us take any measures to restart his heart or breathing should it stop. I spent several minutes at the bedside verifying there were no respirations, no heartbeat, and no blood pressure. In addition, I found his pupils to be fixed and dilated, a sure sign of death.

After answering call lights of several other patients, I informed my charge nurse of Joe's death and eventually sat down at the desk to call his family and update his chart. Although I was still a relatively new nurse this wasn't the first patient death I'd experienced. Yet as I reached for the phone, a small voice in the back of my head said, "Maybe you should double-check before you call them." I don't know why. It wasn't a part of my usual practice to verify death twice before calling family but something urged me to do so. His room was near my desk so I figured, "What the heck?" as I got up and walked back into his room. Just as I stepped toward his bedside he took what is called an agonal breath. It is a deep, ragged, sighing sort of breath, common for someone who is actively dying. However, I wasn't expecting agonal respirations at this point. I was expecting no respirations. Since a phone call to family and physician were at stake, I decided to take my time to be super sure that he had passed. I pulled up a chair so I could take my time to carefully listen for a heartbeat as well as any further respirations. His pupils were still fixed and dilated. Oddly enough over the next five minutes or so his breaths came more frequently and became more regular. A very slow heart beat resumed. Over another five to ten minutes his heart rate and breathing both slowly returned to a normal rate and his pupils slowly returned to normal. I was astounded because I knew he had been dead for at least twenty minutes and possibly as long as ninety. Returning to life at that point was impossible. People don't just die and then come back without extreme medical intervention. And even then it would be impossible to revive an adult who was dead for so long. Yet that's exactly what happened. Moreover, it occurred spontaneously without any intervention on my part. But the most bizarre part was yet to come. After another few minutes he blinked his eyes, looked around the room, then looked at me and said, "Where did they all go?" I had no idea what he was talking about and at the time had not heard about NDEs so I asked what he meant. He then said something about "a crowd of people" having been in his room. Again, I was clueless. Looking back now it all makes sense to me. I know for a fact that he had died and must have exited his body. I now believe that during this time he encountered a group of people or beings of some sort who were there to greet him. But for some reason it was determined that it wasn't quite his "time" yet and so he returned to his body. It's the only way he could have returned and had the brain function required to carry on a conversation after going without oxygen or having a pulse for as long as he did. Additionally, I'm sure that his blood would have been quite acidic at that point and incapable of supporting life or a clear mental state. My only real regret is that I knew nothing about NDEs at the time and didn't think to ask him more about his experience. I did call a family member who laughed it off saying that it sounded like something he would do. As unbelievable as it might have been to read, I documented exactly what happened in his chart and went on with my busy night. He was awake, oriented and perfectly "normal" until he died again (for good) two days later during my days off.

I share this story because it was a first-hand experience in which I witnessed someone die and later return to life without any form of medical intervention which should be medically impossible. He didn't just return to a comatose state as might be expected of one who should have suffered severe brain damage. When he returned he was alert, oriented, verbal, and conversant. I kick myself now for missing the opportunity to learn more about what happened to him. I'm sure there were things he could have told me about where he went, who it was that he saw and why he returned. For me it was a missed opportunity. I share it with you in the hope that you will keep your eyes and ears open so you don't miss any opportunities that come your way. I think events like this are more common than we realize but we blow them off at the time because they don't fit with our view of how the world should be and we are too busy to take the time to sort them out.

Nearing Death Awareness

Nearing death awareness (NDA) is just what it sounds like. It is a term introduced by hospice nurses Maggie Callanan and Patricia Kelley, which conveys the awareness developed by ill patients that tells them death is very near.[14] In some cases it includes certain knowledge about, and sometimes even some control over; the process of dying. However, if loved ones aren't paying attention, they might miss the clues offered by dying patients in the form of odd comments or confusing physical gestures. The loved one's job is to interpret the patient's behavior rather than labeling them as "confused" or over-medicating them in order to "calm" them. Callanan and Kelley noticed these messages from dying patients generally fall into two categories.[15] One is an attempt to describe what they are seeing and experiencing in the process of dying. The other is a request for something they need in order to die more peacefully.

Patients in the first category offer clues that they are seeing or talking with previously deceased loved ones or spiritual beings. They also may know quite specifically when they will die. They are known to use travel language to convey the message that they will be leaving or relocating soon. Examples include talking about the need to find their ticket, pack their suitcase, catch the bus, get in line, catch a flight, and so on.[16] They typically look beyond persons in the room and peer into the right upper corner of the room where they seem to get a glimpse of a world not seen by others. As they look through this open portal to the "other side," dying patients often use words or facial expressions to convey a sense of wonderment, peace, and tranquility or splendor beyond description.

Persons in the second category may wait to die until certain conditions have been met. As a hospital staff nurse, often working with oncology patients I noticed it was not unusual for dying patients to linger far longer than anyone expected. It seemed as if they were waiting for something specific to take place before they could leave. I rarely knew what that something was. However, I couldn't help but notice they sometimes passed shortly after a specific member of the family or long lost friend finally arrived to visit and say "goodbye."

Other authors have also commented on nearing death awareness. Pearson describes subtle transformations in awareness and mood. She also notes the pattern of talking in travel terms within seventy-two hours of death and that patients sometimes even specify the day they will depart.[17] They are nearly always correct. In spite of this, medical practitioners are still sometimes surprised by patients who are expected to live but end up dying after they've seen apparitions of deceased loved ones beckoning to them.

A huge cross-national study of deathbed experiences by psychologists Karlis Osis and Erlendur Haraldsson noted statements alluding to departure among patients not deemed to be terminally ill. Yet, they nearly always proved true.[18] For these reasons, those involved in hospice care have learned to pay attention to such possible signals being sent by their patients. As a result, they often call family members to let them know that death may be near.

Angels

I've heard about angels all my life. Many people claim to believe in them. I've always been inclined to believe, and I noticed they were often mentioned in my readings. Therefore, I began to note descriptive data and trends.

Appearance

The physical appearance of angels varies. This makes sense given that different sources indicate there are many different types of angels. One source reported dozens of types, while another indicated as many as seventy. Descriptions vary also. Some are described as tall as ten feet while others were only four feet in height. Some described long, flowing blond or brown hair while others didn't comment on hair at all. Nearly everyone said they wore long bright, white robes and that they glowed with divine light. Yet some were described in terms of color with bright gold being the most common. However, angels of nearly every color were described by various people.[19]

I suspect you might be wondering about the wings and feathers. Do they or don't they have them? The answer seems to be both. There are many different kinds of angels and so it makes sense to me that their appearance would vary depending upon their type and purpose. Apparently some have wings and feathers and some do not.[20] The features that seemed most impressive for those who claim to have seen them are less tangible but more powerful. These include the projection of a sense of love, peace and serenity. Furthermore their presence always caused the person to feel safe, calm, peaceful, and very loved. In addition, the person may experience pain relief and feel energized.

Purpose

The angels' purpose seems to vary with type. Some provide protection. Others provide a calming presence to relieve fear and anxiety. Yet others provide pain relief. Some relate messages and others take the person on a journey or help them make the transition when they die. I'm sure there are other purposes that I'm unaware of.

They are all messengers of one type or another sent by God to do His work and to help human beings. I haven't yet seen one but I'd certainly like to. They seem to appear most frequently when people are very near death, so I think I will eventually get my chance.

Divine Pain Relief

When patients are near death, a phenomenon that sometimes occurs in the presence of angels is the elimination of pain. This is supported by the patient's own reports and their refusal of pain medication. For example, a young female patient indicated that she was in her last week of life and had over twenty angels in her room twenty-four hours a day to provide comfort from her increasing pain. As her physical condition deteriorated, she felt no discomfort and her mood became more joyful. She attributed it to a "disconnect of her nervous system" as she remained "connected" to the angels and the spiritual world.[21]

While some patients reported their pain was relieved by the presence of angels in their rooms, others reported that angels sometimes took them out of their physical bodies to beautiful places in order to remove them from their physical and emotional pain. For example, one young woman reported being taken to amazing locations around the universe.[22] Another patient, a young boy, described being taken to a beautiful place where he was able to swim with dolphins, seals, penguins, and sometimes other children he had known in the hospital.[23]

Another patient of Dr. Lermas's reported that he began experiencing pain relief when he began conversing with the angels in his room.[24] Also it was pointed out by yet another patient that angels may present themselves at or near the bedside of a dying patient but will not speak unless the patient invites them by speaking first. The communication is in a nonverbal ESP form. The reason the angels wait for an invitation has something to do with their complete respect for our free will.[25]

Sarah

Sarah was an amazing twenty-nine-year-old woman whose emotional and spiritual maturity was far beyond what most people achieve by her age. This may have largely been due to the physical challenges she faced at a young age and the faith and courage with which she responded.

Sarah had been blind since birth because of optic (eye) nerve atrophy. Later, as a young woman, she was diagnosed with an aggressive type of breast cancer. At age twenty-nine she was admitted to hospice for end of life care since chemotherapy was having little effect. [26]

Now as a hospice patient she had the opportunity to share many of her experiences with her physician, Dr. Lerma. He had observed that she exhibited no signs of depression and denied significant pain, rating it as zero to two on the traditional zero to ten pain scale; all in spite of the rapid physical worsening of her condition. She described an interesting correlation between the appearance of angels and disappearance of physical pain, as well as emotional and mental distress. In fact, she stated that "since the angels have been present every day, I have had no physical or emotional pain." She attributed this to the "process of soul detachment from the physical body." She said she accomplished this by "willing the first loving spiritual being [angel] into [her] mind, body, and soul." She added that as more spirits appear, the more quickly the detachment process occurs and the more comfort she experiences.

Pre-death and Deathbed Visions

It is quite common for conscious terminally ill persons who die slowly (rather than suddenly) and are not sedated or are only lightly sedated, to experience visions shortly before death. Such visions have several names including, deathbed visions, pre-death visions, and shared visions. Such visions can occur anywhere from minutes to weeks prior to death, however the vast majority occur within twenty-four hours of death.[27] Observers can become aware that the dying person is having a vision because they begin quietly speaking to an unseen person or are obviously looking toward a specific part of the room. When asked with whom they are speaking, patients typically identify them as deceased loved ones, angels or other spiritual beings. The most commonly identified family member is the deceased mother.[28] The most commonly identified reason for the visit is to relieve the patient's fears and anxiety and to coach them in the crossing over process.[29]

Dr. John Lerma describes dozens of cases of dying patients who experienced pre-death visions. As a board certified hospice and palliative care physician in Texas, he has spent more time at the bedside of dying patients than most doctors ever do. In the process he has learned to observe and listen to them. They have taught him a great deal about the dying process and he shares some of it in his books. His patients describe a wide assortment of visits from deceased loved ones, angels and other spiritual beings. The visits may be as short as a few minutes or as long as several days. There seem to be several purposes to these visits and of course they vary with the individual. Sometimes, with longer visits, patients receive information about what the purpose of their lives has been along with other spiritual information. Shorter visits are usually to provide comfort, relieve anxiety and sometimes to provide instruction about how to cross over. When it's time for the patient to die, the visitor is generally there to coach and assist.

An example described by Osis and Haraldsson is an elderly woman diagnosed with a heart attack. She was conscious, alert, and oriented. She was not taking any sedating medications and had no history of hallucinations. She was quite pleasant and looking forward to a full recovery. Then without notice she reached out her arms and stated that she saw her deceased husband. This caused her to wonder why she hadn't "gone home before." In addition, she commented about the "beautiful place" she saw "with all the flowers and music." She subsequently relaxed into a very serene and peaceful state and died sometime later.[30]

Another comforting trend I've noticed is that when individuals are suffering from some form of lengthy illness and the dying process is prolonged, they are sometimes able to leave their bodies without dying and return intermittently. It typically occurs when they appear to be sleeping very soundly or are semi-comatose and difficult, if not impossible, to arouse. We know this occurs because some patients have reported it and the timing fits within the episodes of very deep sleep. I've wondered if my brother was able to do this. I can't know for sure because he was heavily sedated at the time, but I certainly hope it was true. I like to believe that God may have spared him from much of the trauma that his body endured. I've noticed this pattern in many of my patients as they neared death. Sadly, at the time I wasn't aware of pre-death visions so it didn't occur to me to inquire.

I was rather skeptical when I first read about such visions. Yet as I pondered the matter it began to make sense to me. First, if one accepts the premise that death is not the end and we continue to exist after death, then it is not such a stretch to accept the notion that deceased loved ones might be able to look in on the living from time to time. If they can, then wouldn't they be most likely to do so when they are most needed? Next, if there is a time or place for a portal to open between this world and that one, isn't impending death an obvious time? Finally, as a mother of three I know I would do anything within my power to help my children whether I'm living or dead. This includes helping them cross over when it's their time. Given all of this, a vision where a parent, sibling or other loved one comforts a dying patient and helps them cross over seems quite believable.

The following story is about a personal friend of mine who died of lung cancer several years ago. I feel quite sure that the purpose of his pre-death vision was to alleviate his fear and anxiety so that he could transition peacefully.

Matt

Three years before my own diagnosis I was shocked and saddened to hear about the death of my dear friend Matt, whom I'd known for eighteen years. At one time he lived in my home town, but some years ago he moved to another part of the state. After this I saw him less frequently but we kept in touch by phone and met for dinner and lengthy conversations when he came through town on business. He was a kind and gentle soul and gave the warmest, greatest bear hugs I've ever had.

When I learned that Matt had died of lung cancer I was crushed. He and I had talked many times about his desire to quit smoking. I lost count of the number of attempts he made and always believed one day he would succeed. He didn't tell me about his cancer. I can only guess why, but I suspect he didn't want me to fuss over him. Since I'd never met any of his family nobody notified me when he was ill and dying. Thankfully I learned afterward through another mutual friend.

At his funeral I learned that as Matt was nearing the very end of his life he became quite anxious and restless. This is not uncommon. But I was so relieved and comforted to also learn that he saw a vision of his deceased mother at this time. She appeared at his bedside to convey love and support. I also suspect it was her privilege to help him cross over. From that moment on he was calm and restful and he died within the next twenty-four hours. Upon learning about this I felt more at peace and was so grateful that his mom had been there for him when he needed her.

So Many Angels

In 2004 I was working full-time as a nursing instructor for the local college and also continued to work part-time at the local hospital. One day in the break room, two nurses who were former students of mine struck up a conversation about pre-death visions. As fairly new nurses, neither had had any experiences specific to the topic but were quite curious about a recent terminally ill patient who seemed to be "talking to some unseen person" prior to his death. Since I had recently read several good books on the subject, I too was quite curious. I shared some of the information I had gleaned from the books and we all agreed that "anything is possible" as we ended the conversation and returned to our duties.

Several weeks later when I was back at the hospital in my capacity as Nursing Instructor, Lucy, one of the same nurses from the previous conversation, pulled me aside saying she had something personal she wished to discuss. We arranged to meet on her break a short time later. As we chatted she related that she had recently returned from a three week leave of absence in which she spent time with her dying mother on the East coast. As she sat at her mother's bedside she noticed her mother's mental status fluctuated widely. There were times when she was very tired and weak but awake, oriented and verbal. Then there were other times when she would sleep so soundly as to be nearly comatose. During one of her mom's wakeful times Lucy asked "Where do you go when you are sleeping so soundly?" Her mother responded that she was visiting with her (deceased) mother and her Nana (deceased grandmother) and was "getting ready to join them."

Lucy was surprised but intrigued by her answer and wanted to learn more. So she asked "Did you happen to see any angels?"

Her mom responded with a sleepy smile saying "Oh yes."

Lucy was quite intrigued and inquired once more asking "How many angels did you see mom?"

As her mother fell back to sleep with a smile on her face she whispered "Thousands." She didn't talk further and died within the next twenty-four hours.

Lucy said even though she misses her mother a great deal she feels deeply comforted by the experience and believes her mom is waiting for her with the angels.

Shared Visions

I first became aware of shared visions by reading Glimpses of Eternity by Dr. Raymond Moody and Paul Perry.[33] I've since noticed them in many other books as well, an example being One Last Hug Before I Go by Carla Wills Brandon. They are a form of deathbed vision and are called shared visions because they are simultaneously experienced by two or more people. As Moody points out, when a single person has a vision, others might try to explain it away with various theories about hallucinations, medication side effects or hypoxia (too little oxygen). Even with single-person visions, such arguments don't hold up well. But shared visions are especially significant because when two or more people experience the very same vision, and at least one of them is healthy, the arguments simply fall apart.[34]

Dr. Moody describes several shared death experiences in his book. In the first, he tells of five family members gathered around their dying mother when a bright light suddenly appeared and formed into a portal or opening from the room into another (heavenly) realm. As this occurred some of them looked at one another and one gasped in surprise, indicating they were all seeing the same thing. Next, they heard their mother let out her last breath and then saw her spiritual body rise out of her physical body and exit through the portal. Talking to one another a very short time later, they confirmed they had all seen exactly the same thing and all noted feelings of complete joy.[35]

In another story a woman told Dr. Moody that she sat at her brother's bedside as he was dying of congestive heart failure. He stopped breathing momentarily and she immediately felt the room change shape. Next she felt herself lifted into the air where she felt herself and her brother "swirl around the room as spirits" after which she returned to her own body and normal perspective.[36] Her brother began breathing again and didn't actually die until the next day.

Moody also described a hospice psychologist who describes himself as "not religious" but states that the work he does "has awakened [him] to a spiritual dimension of life." He describes a number of experiences he has had at the bedside of dying patients including the perception of the room changing shape, seeing lights and seeing patients rise out of their physical bodies and move toward structures he saw in the distance (through an open portal).[37]

After-Death Communications

An After-Death Communication, or ADC is a spiritual experience in which a family member or close friend is contacted directly by a deceased loved one. The contact is spontaneous and does not involve rituals, mediums, psychics or the like. According to the ADC website approximately 60 to 120 million Americans have experienced an ADC event at least once.[38] Information at this web site describes numerous types of ADCs including sentient (sensing a presence), auditory (hearing a voice), tactile (feeling a touch), olfactory (smelling a fragrance), visual (seeing a mist, light or the actual person), physical phenomena (blinking lights, electronic devices turning off and on, etc.), symbolic (rainbows, butterflies, etc.), and others.[39] The purpose of the contact isn't always clear but the majority of people interpret it as a reassuring message from the deceased loved one that they are okay and they are happy. A secondary message also conveys the fact that death is not "the end" and that there is more to come for all of us.

A Visit From Rob

Several members of my family and I experienced an ADC the summer of 2010. Ours would most accurately be described as a combination of visual and "other." Those involved included myself, my mother, my daughter-in-law Melissa, and her son Isaac who was a little over two-years-old at the time. This occurred approximately nine months after Rob died. Brad and his family had come from Australia for a five week visit. Isaac and Melissa were visiting with my mother and me at my house.

My mother had been struggling severely to cope with the loss of her first born child, and experienced alternating feelings of sadness, anger, depression, and longing. She was even contemplating moving to Portland, where Rob had lived, in spite of the fact that she no longer had any family and no close friends there. It was I think, a deep desire to be near Rob and somehow thinking she might find comfort in being where he had lived. Rationally I'm sure she knew that she wouldn't find what she was looking for there but was at a loss about how to come to terms with his death.

Reflecting on it later, the whole thing made perfect sense to me. Mom was deeply distressed. Somehow Rob knew this. He didn't want her doing something irrational like moving to a big city where she would be sad and alone. He wanted to find a way to reassure her that he was doing just fine and she needn't worry about him. He recognized his opportunity when he saw little Isaac sitting near her in his high chair contentedly playing with Playdough. What happened next is conveyed in my journal entry below.

Journal August 2010
Isaac Is A Messenger

A few days ago mom, Mel, Isaac, and I were in my living/dining room. Isaac was sitting in the high chair playing with play dough. The rest of us were chatting about something unrelated to Rob. Neither had we mentioned his name or said anything about him.

Suddenly Isaac stopped what he was doing, pointed to a spot just behind and above me and very insistently said "Robbin" several times. Each time he looked at us to see if we understood, then pointed again to the upper right part of the room and repeated himself. It surprised us and we tried to identify what might have triggered this. We kept looking to the area where he was pointing but saw nothing that would have caused him to say Rob's name. We asked Isaac what he was seeing but being two years old with limited verbal skills he was unable to provide a detailed answer. Yet once again and more emphatically than before, he pointed to the same area and said "Yours Robbin," "Yours Robbin," with the emphasis on "yours." He said Rob's name at least eight or ten times and was extremely insistent. It seemed very clear to us that he was seeing something that we could not see. After making his point, Isaac returned to his play dough and never said another word about it.

I believe that Rob paid us a visit that day and since we adults could not see him, Isaac was the messenger. Mom, Mel, and I discussed it later and we had all reached the same conclusion. Sometimes very young children are able to see things that older people do not. Whatever Isaac saw, he was very clear about it and very sure of himself. He had never met Rob and as best we recall, had never uttered Rob's name before or since. Interpret this how you wish, but I firmly believe my brother was in the room that day and the only one that could see him was Isaac. I found it very comforting and so did my mother. In fact, she's finally let go of the idea of moving to Portland. This event helped her understand that Rob is doing just fine and she doesn't need to go looking for him. He can find us anytime he wants to.

Dreams

Dreams don't fall into the same general category as the various sorts of visions I've been describing. Although some dreams I've had could possibly qualify as After-Death-Communications. But since I'm not totally sure, I put them here in the "Dream" category.

Dreams have been attributed profound meaning throughout history. I think one reason they can be so significant is that when we sleep our conscious mind is turned off leaving the unconscious mind in charge. I believe the unconscious mind is more accessible to beings like God or deceased relatives who may wish to send us messages. I'm not talking about the average dreams that most of us have on any given night where we find ourselves naked in public or can't find our high school locker. I'm talking about the ones that are more vivid; the ones that stay with you. Throughout my life, every once in a great, great while, I've had one of those dreams that seems to convey something important that I'm supposed to understand and remember. Since being diagnosed with terminal cancer I've had several.

I had the dream below early in my journey at a time when I was feeling anxious about death and dying. I believe this short but sweet dream was sent to comfort and reassure me; and it did.

Journal September 2010
NDE Dream

Last night I had a dream that I was having an NDE. I felt myself coming close to death (can't explain how I knew, but I did) and I began to see a white light like people talk about. It slowly came closer and closer and got bigger and bigger. It was beautiful and comforting and felt full of love. In my dream I thought, "this is what it will be like when I die." Then I heard a voice (or maybe it was just a thought in my brain) that said something like, "It's not time to die yet, but when it is, it will be ok." Then the light got smaller and went away. When I awoke I remembered the dream and found it to be a great source of comfort.

In the years since my oldest brother died I've had several dreams about him. They've always been brief and the only segment I recall is the one in which he played a part. Yet that brief part was always vivid and memorable. It may be my subconscious messing with my head; or it may be something more. I'm inclined to believe it is something more since they always stick with me and give me comfort.

In one dream I was very ill, near death, and surrounded by family. Though nobody could see him but me, Rob was holding me in his arms throughout the dream and when I died, he was going to carry me over the threshold of death into heaven.

In another dream I was somehow allowed into an area that was just inside heaven's gate or perhaps was a halfway point between this life and that one. I couldn't tell for sure except that I was able to see and converse with people who were deceased. It was a large area with thousands of people (that I could see) but I was aware that it went on and on and that I could see only a small portion of it. I asked to see my brother and after some consideration I was allowed to. He was more joyful than I'd ever seen him in his earthly life and was almost dancing around as he flitted to one person after another. He was so excited to be there and to see everyone that he could barely contain himself and couldn't seem to hold still for more than a minute or two. I was so happy to see him and see how well he was.

At one point I grabbed his arm and said ,"Mom really misses you. Is there anything you would like me to tell her?"

He immediately and joyfully leaned forward, placed his two hands on either side of my face, looked into my eyes, and said, "Tell her I love her!" He said it with more enthusiasm than I can describe. Then with a huge smile on his face he danced away to greet other people.

In every dream he has been youthful (probably in his thirties), extremely healthy, at peace, and happier than he'd ever been in his life. Were they just dreams? Maybe. But they were comforting and did my heart good. I've shared them with my mother and other family who also seem to take comfort in them. In their own way they cause me to look forward to the day that I am allowed to cross over and be united with Rob, Matt, and others that I miss. Will I miss the ones I leave behind? I cannot say for sure how I will feel when I'm in heaven but it is difficult to imagine not missing them. However, my great comfort will be knowing that I will have the honor of greeting them one day soon when it's their turn to cross over.

The end is just another beginning.

Being diagnosed with a fatal disease rocked my world. It stopped me dead in my tracks and forced me to reevaluate everything about my life including how I was spending my time and who I was spending it with. It also forced me to accept the reality that my time here is very limited. Until then, I realized I had been living under the illusion that there would always be more time. And now I know, really know, that it's just not true. I have today. I have now. And that's all I know for sure, so I need to be thoughtful about how I spend it. Whether it's a quiet day resting alone at home, or watching my grandkids play soft ball, or calling loved ones who live far away, I now spend my time in a more intentional way.

Though I'd always been a believer, my faith has deepened. While I don't attend church any more often, I am more intentional about my time with God. I converse with Him much more frequently, trying to avoid the shallow "gimme, gimme" prayers of the past. Instead I (mostly) remember to pray from faith, rather than fear. When I do, I've noticed that I feel a deeper sense that the answer will come and so I more eagerly look forward to seeing it. When I do pray for things, rather than giving God a "wish list," I'm more likely to make requests like, "What do you want me to learn from this? Please help me understand how I can better support (name of person in need). Please help me to hear you more clearly," and, "Please help me fulfill your purpose for me today." And I try to remember to thank Him for his answers. I'm also more likely to remember to thank Him for His goodness, grace, mercy and love.

I continue to find support in the writings of others. I've always enjoyed reading but I read even more now than before. I still enjoy novels, adventure stories and mysteries. But now I'm more likely to read books of a spiritual nature, books about end-of-life issues, and those that challenge me to think, learn, and grow. I enjoy how all of these books challenge me to think about things in new and different ways, all of which helps me as I continue my spiritual journey.

As you've probably noticed, my faith has a great impact on my coping ability. I realize that many people on this planet live and die without any particular sort of faith. Yet I cannot imagine how they do this. I need hope like I need the air that I breathe. And my faith gives me so many reasons to hope.

Now I do realize that I may have some parts of it all wrong. Consequently, I may be in for some surprises when I pass to "the other side." In fact, it seems inevitable. But I'm okay with that. What I do have is a belief system that feels grounded and safe. And when I have difficult days or moments of fear, I wrap it around me like a beautiful, warm quilt and know that I am loved.

Epilogue

As I put the finishing touches on this book, it is the spring of 2017. It's been a rich journey full of twists and turns, ups and downs. And I couldn't possibly feel more thankful than I do for the "extra" time God has given me and the many lessons I've learned.

Some wonderful changes have taken place in my life during this time. I've had the joy of being closely involved in my first granddaughter's life. Already five years old she is a never-ending source of great joy. My daughter keeps her eyes on me and does nearly all of the cooking to make sure I eat something besides cold cereal and chocolate Ensure. I've done so well in that regard that I managed to locate the twenty pounds I lost after chemotherapy plus another twenty I wasn't really looking for. While I'm not worried about it I do hope to not "find" anymore.

In August of 2015 my oldest son and his wife gave me one of the best surprises of my life by moving their family to the States. In fact, they and their four boys now live a mere ten-minute drive from me. What a joy it has been to have them so close and to have the opportunity to get to know my grandsons in a much deeper way.

Last but certainly not least, my middle son Brian and his wife produced my fifth grandson the summer of 2015 plus my sixth grandson and second granddaughter (twins!) in early 2016. So my life is very full and has become busier than I ever expected given my early "retirement." I'd not dared to dream I would live long enough to see and hold my first granddaughter, not to mention living long enough to have eight grandchildren (and their parents) all living nearby. God has been good!

I continue to see my oncologist, Dr. Shell, every three months and undergo CT and bone scans every six months. I never achieved official "remission," but the cancer seemed to be in a steady holding pattern for several years which provided a gift of "time" I shall forever be grateful for. In addition, my cancer status remained essentially unchanged for nearly another two years in spite of me taking no cancer treatment at all for that time. What a blessing that was! As time passed my body slowly returned to a state of near-normalcy. Unfortunately my normal energy level never returned but in most other respects I felt almost like my old self again.

As of now it's been seven years since my initial diagnosis in May, 2010, and I've lived at least six years longer than I ever expected to. During this time I was well aware that my condition could change significantly at any time. This knowledge kept me humble and grateful and reminded me to live in the moment, savoring the now as fully as possible.

Then, on the morning of this past New Year's Eve I got out of bed and collapsed on the floor as my left hip totally gave out on me. The pain was beyond anything I had yet experienced. I had recently noticed a slow worsening of pain in that hip. I (and my doctor) both thought it was a worsening of arthritis or possibly bursitis, both being inflammatory conditions that are treatable. The pain had been annoying but not severe. In fact we had just chatted about it the previous Thursday and devised a plan for me to be evaluated by an orthopedic physician. She also sent me directly to Radiation/ Oncology that very day for evaluation and possible treatment. Sadly, I learned there that the cancer had taken up residence in one of the main bones that comprises my left hip socket and had eroded completely through it. Consequently any weight-bearing or active motion of that leg caused severe pain. It is probably not operable so immediate treatment included increased pain medications and a five-day course of radiation to the involved bone. In the meantime my daughter picked up a walker, a shower chair, and handheld shower for me. It so happens that my brother Rick works at a medical supply store in town. So between the two of them, they knew what sort of equipment I was going to need around the house. Because pain was more of an issue now I sought a palliative care consultation. Unfortunately our town is currently between palliative care physicians. The new one arrives in July. But the palliative care nurse Ginny, has been awesome! She acts similarly to a case manager with a focus on pain and symptom management. She is good at identifying my needs, finding ways to meet them and advocates for me with other members of the health care team (especially the doctors). I really can't say enough great things about her but for now, this will have to suffice.

So the past few months have been a flurry of appointments, evaluations, consultations and tests. I resumed the Tarceva at the lower dose I'd last been on and seemed to tolerate it ok for about two months. Then all hell broke loose in my GI tract much as it had back when I had to discontinue the Taceva several years ago. Only this time it was actually worse and occurred three separate times two of which occurred after I had stopped Tarceva. On one such occasion I ended up in the emergency room. I had become severely dehydrated in just four to five hours with severe, watery diarrhea, severe vomiting, and no ability to retain any sort of liquids or oral medications. I was grateful to have Nicole and mom in the house for the next couple of weeks to look after the dogs and keep bringing me liquids. My gut was so touchy that I was afraid to eat solid food. But over the next month I slowly transitioned back to a fairly normal diet. I've had no further episodes.

Since I'd discontinued the Tarceva I had expected my next scan to show bad news. In fact I'd decided to ask my doctor about a hospice referral. But she and I were both surprised at how good the scan looked. Not that I'm healed mind you, but it did show some actual improvement. I didn't think two months on the Tarceva was long enough to provide much of a difference. But it did. The tumor area in my hip had visibly shrunk. I have no idea how long this improvement will last, but I'm grateful for it and plan to enjoy every minute I get.

God continues to remind me that this journey is all about trust, gratitude, faith, and love. Some days it feels easy. Some days are more challenging. Yet I know my final destination is heaven and I will not be traveling alone. And while there may be more some bumps and bruises ahead, I know God's mercy and grace will guide me each step of the way.

Recommended Reading

◘ Near Death Experiences (NDEs)

֍ About Angels

≑ After-Death Communications / After-Death Encounters
(ADCs & ADEs)

√ Heaven Visited, Described

* Visions (deathbed, predeath, shared, etc.)

𝑥 *Hope Affirming*

☼ Palliative Care and/or Hospice

§ *Faith Affirming*

♠ Personal Favorite

Research-Based Data

Q Transformative Effects

◘ √ ♠ Alexander, Eben. *Proof of Heaven: A Neurosurgeon's Journey into the Afterlife*. Simon & Schuster. 2012.

√ Alexander, Eben. *The Map of Heaven: How Science, Religion, and Ordinary People Are Proving the Afterlife*. Simon & Schuster. Kindle Edition. Copyright © 2014 by Eben Alexander LLC.

♦ § Anderson, Reggie. *Appointments with Heaven: The True Story of a Country Doctor's Healing Encounters with the Hereafter.* Tyndale Momentum. Kindle edition. Copyright © 2013 by Reggie Anderson.

♦ ⚖ * # Arcangel, Dianne, *Afterlife Encounters: Ordinary People, Extraordinary Experiences.* Hampton Roads Publishing Company Inc. Charlottesville, VA. 2005, © by Dianne Arcangel.

◻ Atwater, P.M.H., *I Died Three Times in 1977 - The Complete Story.* Kindle Edition. Cinema of the Mind / Starving Artists Workshop. E-Published by Starving Artists Workshop . © 2010 P.M.H. Atwater.

◻ Atwater, P.M.H, *The Big Book of Near Death Experiences: The Ultimate Guide to What Happens When We Die.* Hampton Roads Publishing Inc. 2007.

◻ ♦ Beam, Christy Wilson, *Miracles From Heaven: A Little Girl and Her Amazing Story of Healing.* © 2015, Christy Wilson Beam. Hachette Book Groups, Inc., New York, N.Y.

◻ Bellg MD, Laurin. *Near Death in the ICU: Stories from Patients Near Death and Why We Should Listen to Them.* Sloan Press. Kindle Edition. © 2016. Appleton, WI.

◻ Black, Capt. Dale; Ken Gire. *Flight to Heaven: A Plane Crash...A Lone Survivor...A Journey to Heaven--and Back.* Baker Publishing Group, © 2010. Kindle Edition.

◻ √ Brinkley, Dannion with Paul Perry. *Saved by the Light: The True Story of a Man Who Died Twice and the Profound Revelations He Received.* Harper Paperbacks, a division of Harper Collins Publishers, 1994 by Villard Books. © 1994 Dannion Brinkley with Paul Perry.

◻ √ ♦ Burpo, Todd, Colton Burpo, Lynn Vincent. *Heaven is For Real: A Little Boy's Astounding Story of His Trip to Heaven and Back.* Harper Collins Christian Publishing: Thomas Nelson, 2011.

♠ Byock, Ira. *Dying Well: Peace and Possibilities at the end of Life.* Riverhead books. 1998.

* ♠ Callanan, Maggie. *Final Journeys: A Practical Guide for Bringing Care and Comfort at the End of Life.* 2009.

* ♠ Callanan, Maggie, and Patricia Kelley. *Final Gifts: Understanding the Special Awareness, Needs, and Communications of the Dying.* New York: Bantam, 1992.

DeMoss, Nancy Leigh with Lawrence Kimbrough. *Choosing Gratitude: Your Journey to Joy.* 2009 Moody Publishers, Chicago.

√ Dyer, Dr. Wayne W. and Dee Garnes. *Memories of Heaven: Children's Astounding Recollections of the Time Before They Came to Earth.* Hay House, Inc. © 2015, Kindle Edition.

𝓍 ♠ Fanslow-Brunjes, Cathleen. *Using the Power of Hope to Cope with Dying: The Four Stages of Hope.* Quill Driver Books, an imprint of Lind Publishing © 2008. Fresno, CA.

𝓍 ♠ Frankl, Sara and Mary Carver. *Choose Joy: Finding Hope and Purpose When Life Hurts.*

Frankl, Victor E. *Man's Search for Meaning.* Beacon Press, 1949, 1992, Boston, MA

√ Gaulden, Ed. *Heaven, A Joyful Place: A true, visit to Heaven*, story Ed Gaulden July 2012 Revised July 2013, Kindle edition.

♠ Gawande, Atul. *Being Mortal: Medicine and What Matters in the End.* Metropolitan Books. Henry Holt & Company. 2014.

◘ Goodwin, Celeste and Matthew. *A Boy Back From Heaven.* Cedar Fort, Inc.. Kindle Edition. © 2014 Celeste and Matthew Goodwin

𝓍 ♠ Groopman, Jerome. *The Anatomy of Hope: How People Prevail in the Face of Illness.* NY: Random House, 2005.

Groves, Richard F. and Henriette Ann Klauser, *The American Book of Living and Dying: Lessons in Healing Spiritual Pain.* Celestial

Arts, an imprint of Crown Publishing Group, a division of Random House, Inc., New York. 2005, 2009.

Guggenheim Bill and Jill Guggenheim, *Hello From Heaven: a New Field of Research, After-Death Communication Confirms that Life and Love are Eternal.* Bantam Books, New York © 1995.

* # Haraldsson Ph.D, Erlendur; Osis Ph.D, Karlis. *At the Hour of Death: A New Look at Evidence for Life After Death.* White Crow Books. Kindle Edition. Copyright © 2012 by Erlendur Haraldsson.

ϰ * ☼ ⸎ Harris, Trudy. *Glimpses of Heaven: True Stories of Hope & Peace at the End of Life's Journey.* Grand Rapids, MI: Revell a division of Baker Publishing Group, 2008.

ϰ * ☼ ⸎ Harris, Trudy. *More Glimpses of Heaven: Inspiring True Stories of Hope & Peace at the End of Life's Journey.* Grand Rapids, MI: Revell a division of Baker Publishing Group, 2010.

⸎ Hayden, L. C. *Angels Around Us.* Kindle Edition, © 2011 by L. C. Hayden.

Keane, Colm. *We'll Meet Again.* Penguin Books Ltd. Kindle Edition. Copyright © Colm Keane, 2013.

* ⸎ Kessler, David. *Visions, Trips and Crowded Rooms: Who and What You See Before You Die.* Carlsbad, CA: Hay House, 2010.

* Koedam, Ineke. *In the Light of Death: Experiences on the threshold between life and death.* White Crow Productions Ltd. Kindle Edition. © 2015.

Kübler-Ross, Elisabeth. *On Death and Dying: What the Dying Have to Teach Doctors, Nurses, Clergy & Their Own Families.* Scribner © 2014. Kindle Edition.

* ⸎ ☼ ⸎ Lerma, John. *Into the Light: Real Life Stories About Angelic Visits, Visions of the Afterlife, and Other Pre-Death Experiences.* Franklin Lakes, NJ: New Page Books, a division of the Career Press. Kindle Edition 2007.

* ⚛ ☼ ♪ Lerma, John. *Learning from the Light: Pre-Death Experiences, Prophecies, and Angelic Messages of Hope.* Kindle Edition. Career Press 2009, © Dr. John Lerma.

◘ Lund, Sharon; Hector Keaopa'uhane; Monica Hagen. *There Is More . . . 18 Near-Death Experiences* (Sacred Life Series). Sacred Life Publishers 2010. Kindle Edition.

◘ Malarkey, Kevin. *The Boy Who Came Back from Heaven: A Remarkable Account of Miracles, Angels, and Life beyond This World.* Tyndale House Publishers. Kindle Edition. © 2010 Kevin Malarkey.

◘ Maltby, Deirdre Dewitt. *While I Was Out...: My Near-Death Experience & Soul Altering Journey.* Xlibris US. © 2012, Kindle Edition.

◘ ♪ Moody, Raymond. *Life After Life: The Investigation of a Phenomenon-Survival of Bodily Death.* Harper One, 2015.

Moody, Raymond. *The Light Beyond: New Exploration by the Author of Life After Life.* Raymond A. Moody, Jr. 2011.

◘ Moody, Raymond Jr. MD, *Reflections on Life After Life: More Important Discoveries in the Ongoing Investigation of Survival of Life After Bodily Death*, Bantam/Mockingbird Books, 2011.

* ♪ Moody, Raymond Jr. MD. With Paul Perry, *Glimpses of Eternity: Sharing a Loved One's Passage from this Life to the Next.* New York: Guideposts, 2010.

◘ Moorjani, Anita. *Dying to be Me: My Journey from Cancer, to Near Death, to True Healing.* CA: Hay House, 2012.

◘ ⓠ Mumford, Nigel W. D., *Dying to Live: How Near Death Experiences Transform Our Faith.* Koehler Studios, Inc.2016, Kindle Edition. © Copyright 2016, Nigel W. D. Mumford.

◘ ⚛ ♪ Neal, Mary. *To Heaven and Back: A Doctor's Extraordinary Account of Her Death, Heaven, Angels, and Life Again, a True Story.* Colorado Springs, CO: Mary C. Neal, 2012.

§ ♋ Norris, Kathleen, *Amazing Grace: A Vocabulary of Faith*. Riverhead Books, N.Y. 1998.

§ ♋ Nouwen, Henri J. M., *With Open Hands*. Ave Maria Press, Notre Dame Indiana. © 1975, 1995, 2005.

◘ Olsen, Jeff with Lee Nelson. *I Knew Their Hearts: The Amazing True Story of a Journey Beyond the Vein and Learning the Silent Language of the Heart*. Cedar Fort: 2012.

◘ Parti, Rajiv, MD with Paul Perry. *Dying to Wake Up: A Doctor's Voyage into the Afterlife and the Wisdom He Brought Back*. Atria Books, An Imprint of Simon & Schuster, Inc. New York, 2016.

χ Pedersen, Laura Frankl and Choose Joy Foundation.com. *Choose Surrender: a Blog by Laura Pedersen*. New York, © 2016 by the Sara "Gitz" Frankl Memorial Foundation.

◘ * Pearson, Patricia. *Opening Heaven's Door: Investigating Stories of Life, Death, and What Comes After*. Atria Books and Simon & Schuster: 2014.

◘ Don Piper; Cecil Murphey. *90 Minutes in Heaven: A True Story of Death & Life*. Kindle Edition. Murphy-Revell, 2004.

◘ Ritchie, George G. and Elizabeth Sherrill. *Return from Tomorrow*. Baker Publishing Group. Kindle Edition. © 1978, 2007 by George G. Ritchie. Published by Chosen Books A division of Baker Publishing Group.

√ Roberts, Christopher. *Heaven: My Testimony About Life In Heaven* (Miraculous Book 1). Kindle Edition. © 2014 Christopher Roberts. U.S.A.

◘ ꧁ Roberts, Patti. *I Believe, Book I: Real People's Stories, Thoughts & Beliefs about Guardian Angels, Heaven, Soul Mates, The Afterlife, Near Death*. Compiled and published by Patti Roberts, 2011.

Acknowledgments

Every author has a team of people that have guided, coached and cheered them on through the process of writing, editing and publication. I am no exception and owe a great debt of gratitude to the ladies at She Writes Press.

About the Author

Sharon Eagle and her five siblings were raised in the beautiful Willamette Valley in western Oregon. After high school, Eagle left home to attend college in southern Idaho but withdrew during her second year, feeling unsure of her life goals. Over the next ten years, she relocated to central Washington, married, and had three children. While they were still quite young, she discovered her interest in health care and entered the nursing program at the local college. She began her career working the night shift at the town's only hospital. She discovered her love of teaching when students from the local nursing program came to the hospital for their clinical rotations. That inspired her to earn a master's degree that would qualify her to teach nursing on a full-time basis. During the last several years of her career, she authored a number of health care textbooks. Her career, which lasted a total of twenty-four years, ended prematurely when she was diagnosed with lung cancer. Eagle is a mother of three and a grandmother of eight (including twins) and, when time and energy permit, loves to read and quilt.

SELECTED TITLES FROM SHE WRITES PRESS

She Writes Press is an independent publishing company
founded to serve women writers everywhere.
Visit us at www.shewritespress.com.

From Sun to Sun: A Hospice Nurse's Reflection on the Art of Dying by Nina
Angela McKissock $16.95, 978-1-63152-808-8
Weary from the fear people have of talking about the process of dying
and death, a highly experienced registered nurse takes the reader into
the world of twenty-one of her beloved patients as they prepare to leave
this earth.

The Space Between: A Memoir of Mother-Daughter Love at the End of Life
by Virginia A. Simpson $16.95, 978-1-63152-049-5
When a life-threatening illness makes it necessary for Virginia Simpson's
mother, Ruth, to come live with her, Simpson struggles to heal their relationship before Ruth dies.

Renewable: One Woman's Search for Simplicity, Faithfulness, and Hope by
Eileen Flanagan $16.95, 978-1-63152-968-9
At age forty-nine, Eileen Flanagan had an aching feeling that she wasn't
living up to her youthful ideals or potential, so she started trying to change
the world—and in doing so, she found the courage to change her life.

*Warrior Mother: A Memoir of Fierce Love, Unbearable Loss, and Rituals
that Heal* by Sheila K. Collins, PhD. $16.95, 978-1-938314-46-9
The story of the lengths one mother goes to when two of her three adult
children are diagnosed with potentially terminal diseases.

This Trip Will Change Your Life: A Shaman's Story of Spirit Evolution by
Jennifer B. Monahan $16.95, 978-1-63152-111-9
One woman's inspirational story of finding her life purpose and the messages and training she received from the spirit world as she became a
shamanic healer.

Four Funerals and a Wedding: Resilience in a Time of Grief by Jill Smolowe
$16.95, 978-1-938314-72-8
When journalist Jill Smolowe lost four family members in less than two
years, she turned to modern bereavement research for answers—and
made some surprising discoveries.